A DOCTOR'S VISITS

A DOCTOR'S VISITS

Ian M Brown

Regards

1 Nov 04

Ian

The Book Guild Ltd
Sussex, England

First published in Great Britain in 2003 by
The Book Guild Ltd
25 High Street
Lewes, East Sussex
BN7 2LU

Copyright © Dr Ian M Brown 2003

The right of Dr Ian M Brown to be identified as the author of
this work has been asserted by him in accordance with the
Copyright, Designs and Patents Act 1988.

All rights reserved. No part of this publication may be reproduced,
transmitted, or stored in a retrieval system, in any form or by any means,
without permission in writing from the publisher, nor be otherwise circulated
in any form of binding or cover other than that in which it is published and
without a similar condition being imposed on the subsequent purchaser.

Typesetting in Times by
Acorn Bookwork, Salisbury, Wiltshire

Printed in Great Britain by
Antony Rowe Ltd, Chippenham, Wiltshire

A catalogue record for this book is available from
The British Library.

ISBN 1 85776 693 8

To my wife, Helen

CONTENTS

PART ONE

Early Days	3
North Africa – June 1943	17
Italy – April 1944	22

PART TWO

Italian Campaign – August 1944	35
Venice	39
Post-War	52
B.M.A.	74
Medical Administration	83
A Précis of the History of the Medical Superintendent's society	87
Holland	93
Belgium – May 1962	95
Serre Chevalier – 1962	99
Denmark – 1963	105
Israel – November 1964	109
Sweden – June 1965	115
Portugal – 1965	117

Finland – June 1966	122
Norway – 1966	127
Jugoslavia	129
North America – August 1967	132
Germany, Dusseldorf – June 1969	137
Dublin – June 1971	140
Russia – 1972	146
Canada – 1973	159
Jamaica – April 1974	165
Majorca – 1975	168
Japan – 1979–80	171
A Lightning Tour of Europe	177
Christmas in Rome – December 1984	179
France	183
Paris	189
The Auvergne – 1968	197
The Vosges – 1971	202
Rabelais	214
The War Leaders	219
Misunderstandings	234
Words of the Great	235
Fire-Eaters	236
Hobbies	237
Gaugin	252

Family Life	256
Conclusions	258
Bibliography	260

PART ONE

EARLY DAYS

For some, childhood memories and happy schooldays provide pleasurable recollections, but my enjoyment of life has grown progressively during the last 70 years, each year being more stimulating and exciting. This does not imply criticism of life at home and school, which was austere and, by its very austerity, made me yearn for a better life.

Formal education was at Robert Gordon's College, Aberdeen, founded by an Aberdeen man who became a successful merchant in Danzig, and the school provided education for many boys who later held prominent positions in many parts of the world. The London Gordonians have an annual dinner and the last I attended was held in the House of Lords. We were then told of Lord Hailsham, Lord Chancellor, resplendent in wig and robe, greeting Neil Kinnock with a stentorian shout of 'Neil', at which a visiting group from overseas obsequiously knelt down.

Each year we had a school photograph, with several hundred boys assembled in four tiers, the photographer using a slowly revolving camera to get the best results rather than take a still photograph from a greater distance. One bright lad positioned himself at the right side on the front row and, whilst the camera was slowly moving round, ran behind the assembled boys to take a seat at the left side, so he appeared twice in the same photograph.

An excellent tuition gave me an abiding interest in the classics as well as scientific subjects. A classical education is now sometimes decried but I can still recite in Latin a Horatian ode which I remember clearly 70 years later. Roughly translated it means: 'By my writings, I have erected a monument more lasting than bronze or the thrones of kings, higher than the pyramids, which neither the bitter wind or impotent seas can destroy. Nor can the countless years or passage of time ...' and so on.

Later I gained a great deal from an interest in the Boy Scout movement, which taught me to be self-sufficient. As a Boy Scout I learned all sorts of useful skills for which badges were awarded. Amongst others, I had a cook's badge. To qualify for this the boy had to light a fire and cook a 'damper' – a form of pancake which tasted rather as its name suggested.

On the morning when I was due to set off to take the cook's badge examination, I decided to carry the flour required in an Andrews' Liver Salts tin. Now it so happened that we had in the bathroom cabinet a new nearly full tin and a second tin which was almost empty. So I tipped the balance of the nearly empty tin into the new container and filled the empty tin with flour. Unfortunately I took the wrong tin. Lighting the fire was easy, but when I poured water on to my 'flour' in the billycan, it frothed up and extinguished the fire in a way that would have gladdened the heart of an experienced fireman. But I managed to borrow some flour from one of my fellow competitors and passed the test. Then came the cyclist badge, the sewing badge, the pathfinder badge, the first aid badge and so on until I became a First Class Scout with a King's Scout badge and All Round Cords.

This made me feel really good, as it must have done to the thousands of others who achieved the same thing.

Scout camps were highlights of my early life and expeditions on a push-bike with pannier bags on the back carrying a tent, cooking utensils etc., took me down as far as the Lake District. I can still remember our longest day – Glasgow to Carlisle – about 100 miles, I think.

Good fortune resulted in a place in a university bursary competition so that with the help given, and a grant from the Carnegie Trust, I was able to start medical school at the early age of 16.

The gap between leaving school and starting university was filled by getting a job as a cabin-boy in a 500-ton coal boat, plying from Aberdeen to Blyth in Northumberland, loading there with coal and delivering to Le Tréport near Dieppe in Northern France.

My duties included polishing the brass binnacle and bridge rails as well as climbing a steel ladder up the funnel to polish the brass siren. The cleaning material was a mixture of colsa oil and bathbrick, contained in a tin with a wire handle, and applied with a piece of waste rag. It was at times disconcerting to be at the top of the funnel and look down straight into the sea below when the ship rolled. The ship was run by the mate, a small wizened quick-witted man, who was well aware that the skipper drank at least a bottle of whisky a day, but the pair seemed to get on well together. My bunk was in the locker room and as I rolled over in bed at night, my elbows would knock on the partition on the other side of which was the mate's bunk. So every night, he would shout out, 'Stop haimmerin' on the bulkheed' as if I were doing it on purpose.

After loading coal at Blyth, the whole vessel was covered in coal dust, but by the time we reached Le Tréport things were more or less ship-shape.

My first visit to France was particularly fascinating, enabling me to practice my schoolboy French. The only admonition given me by the skipper before going ashore was, 'Look out for these bloody geraniums.' In fact there seemed to be only one gendarme in the small port and he was most helpful, as were the *sapeurs-pompiers* – the fire brigade – who proudly showed me their fire station.

Life at university was hard work for me, with little pleasure. Pocket money was scarce – I would walk three miles to the university rather than spend one and a half-penny on a tram fare. It was possible to supplement one's income by postal sorting at Christmas, working for 18 hours at a stretch for the peak period; grouse beating on the moors was a healthy way of earning a little extra in summer. Whilst at university I joined the Officer Training Corps. This involved weekly drills – including stretcher drill – and annual camps. In 1938, I was promoted to the rank of Lance Corporal and, with one other cadet to represent Aberdeen, went to Aldershot for a two-week course. As every university OTC had a different uniform we presented a strange sight when we were marched about the different military establishments. Nothing happened to suggest that a war was imminent.

One lecture which I can clearly recall dealt with Boys anti-tank guns – modified pea shooters.

'Of course these Continental armies believe in tanks, but we know – we know with certainty – that we can knock them out with ease. Much too vulnerable.'

Our lecturer, booted and spurred, was full of confidence. He spoke well but we never found out whether or not he was able to write.

Unfortunately, I developed tonsillitis one evening, although most of my tonsils had been removed under chloroform by my uncle who operated on the kitchen table, when I was about four or five years of age.

In the Aldershot M.I. Room, the duty orderly handed me a Winchester quart bottle of Mist. Alba and said, 'Take a swig of that after shaking the bottle.'

It seemed that the tumblers were locked up.

Next day I was admitted to the Cambridge Military Hospital, Aldershot and treated with the new wonder drug Prontosil Rubrum, developed by the German firm of Bayer during research into dyestuffs. It was the first of the sulpho-namides – a later version was manufactured in Great Britain by May and Baker – and called M. and B. 693.

We were all urged to join the regular army after qualifying in medicine and some of those present seemed to like the idea.

There was obviously quite a bit of the Maginot Line attitude prevalent and not much forward thinking as far as we could determine.

During the previous year, in August 1937, the then Home Secretary, Sir Samuel Hoare, spoke to an audience of boys at the Public Schools' Aviation Camp, Mousehold, Norwich, saying, 'The equipment of the British defence services and the organisation for producing armaments on a large scale are so highly efficient today that it is most unlikely that any country would consider involving itself in a war against us.'

He referred to the comparative suddenness with which submarines and aircraft were introduced as effective weapons of attack and said that the rapid progress in recent years in defensive measures made one wonder whether this generation would see defence weapons reach the same state of efficiency as the weapons of attack.

Instancing the improved armaments of battleships, Sir Samuel said the development of guns capable of sustaining concentrated anti-aircraft fire was such that a massed dive on a battleship would probably result in at least ten enemy aircraft being brought down.

It seemed likely that in the future attackers would not consider battleships a worthwhile target, but would concentrate on more strategic objects where there was less risk of loss to the attackers.

Sir Samuel described the latest developments in the defence of the civil population against gas and incendiary bombs by the distribution of gas-masks to all sections of the population from babyhood to old age. There would also be available, he said, a large supply of cheap fire extinguishers to cope with the many fires that might easily occur.

Foresight is a rare commodity.

When I lecture on how things change in 100 years, I make a simple drawing on the blackboard:

1902   PAWNSHOPS   O
                                    O   O

2002   PORNSHOPS   ⊙   ⊙

Who could have forecast such change?

After obtaining 'Certificate B' from the Officer Training Corps, I received a document implying that it would entitle me to a degree of seniority if ever I were to serve in the army. When I presented the paper after being called up, I formed the impression from the colourful language of the orderly room sergeant that it would be of use only for personal hygiene.

When I was a Boy Scout I had got to know Ian Buchan, then a qualified pharmacist. He was unhappy where he was, apprenticed to a rather tyrannical boss, so I persuaded him to give this up and start medical school with me. Ian Buchan and I became good friends from then on and I can still recall climbing in the Cairngorms and getting to the summit of Ben Macdhui (4,300 ft.) in a snowstorm on New Year's Day.

We had set off from Maggie Gruer's bothy at Inverey after cycling the 60 miles or so up Deeside from Aberdeen. Dressed in Officers Training Corps greatcoats and army boots, we were ill-fitted to climb mountains in the prevailing weather, but fortunately one of the party, Fraser Ross, had been a surveyor in Nigeria before going to medical school and could read a compass, otherwise we would have perished. We got down the icy slopes on our behinds, holding up our legs with our hands clasped between our knees. What would have happened if we had struck a rock during the descent?

The fact that Ian Buchan was a qualified pharmacist and that I had won the Strachan Bursary in Clinical Medicine and Therapeutics in June 1940, enabled us to apply for the two resident clinical assistant posts at the Aberdeen Royal Mental Hospital. These were much sought after posts because they provided free board and lodging for one year, in return for doing the dispensing for 1,000 patients, carrying out clinical procedures such as lumbar punctures, tube-feeding and so on, and at the same time continuing studies at the medical school.

I can clearly remember my first night there. After arriving at about 7.00 p.m. I was told that I had to do a post-mortem – something I had never done before. The porters were off duty, so I was given a huge key and directed in the dark to the mortuary which stood on its own in the grounds.

The patient had died of a volvulus – a twisted intestine – and I had to do the whole exercise single-handed. This is what it means to be thrown in at the deep end.

We had as our bedroom a former patients' cell with spy hole and self-locking door. The dining room we shared with the deputy medical superintendent, Dr Raitt, plus a psychiatrist who used to study a newspaper upside down, another Glaswegian who enjoyed a wee dram. The room was cockroach-ridden, so that when we came in late and switched on the light, they would scuttle away out of sight (the cockroaches, not the medical staff).

Every day, early in the morning, we had to go round tube-feeding the patients if required, then start the dispensing. Our first job was to clear out the debris left by our predecessors – and I mistakenly jettisoned a bottle marked Vin Xeres – which I later learned was sherry. It was wartime, 1940, and paraldehyde was issued with the agreement that the nursing staff could administer this without medical authority if the air-raid sirens were to sound. How we hated the sound of the sirens – not because of the occasional bombs – but because we knew that the following morning we would have to dispense scores of bottles of paraldehyde.

We dispensed jam jars containing Virol and Ostomalt, which were stored in metal drums with taps at the bottom end. In the cold weather, both substances were viscous and flowed very slowly into the jam jars and we were accustomed to getting on with making up powders, mixtures and so on whilst the jars slowly filled up. Unfortunately, on one occasion, we left the dispensary, forgetting to turn off the Virol and Ostomalt taps. Quite apart from the waste of good material, it was no fun cleaning up a dispensary floor one inch deep in Virol and Ostomalt. Of course it was more than our jobs were worth to report the matter to the domestic supervisor who could have arranged to clean the floor.

Another mishap occurred after I had asked the hospital carpenter to section off a flat drawer which held labels 'Shake the bottle', 'Poison', 'For external use only' etc. We had methodically sorted out all the labels and placed them in their own compartments in the drawer when I inadvertently pulled the drawer out of its recess and the whole collection of labels fluttered to the floor. Most people react to such happenings by uttering some expletive. One of the many peculiar aspects of my behaviour is that I never swear. Certainly I do not regard this as some sign of moral rectitude, but simply feel that one ought to be able to express one's reactions in some more sophisticated way. A much worse facet of my character is that I am inclined to use violence when I feel that a wrongful act has been committed, but fortunately have never been provoked to do so.

In the mental hospital we had to learn to tolerate abuse and violence. And we British are a tolerant, perhaps too tolerant, race. Mental abnormality, including senile decay, is often put forward as a pardonable reason for some forms of outrageous behaviour.

But life was at times amusing. At the back gate, the street led to the local slaughterhouse. One sunny afternoon, a herd of bullocks was being driven for slaughter when one turned aside, entered the back gate and actually got into a ward. The sister in charge shut herself in a linen cupboard, so that it was a patient called Lizzie who telephoned for help.

When the call came to the doctors' sitting room where we were having tea I answered the phone and said to Dr Raitt, 'Lizzie says that there is a bullock in her ward.'

'What! Lizzie again. She comes out with the most fantastic things at times.'

However, he sent me to investigate and by the time I arrived in the ward, the drover had come in and taken charge of the animal. All the patients were terrified with one exception, Little Jeannie.

'We've had lions and tigers roaming this ward for as long as I can remember, so a bullock certainly wouldn't frighten me.'

Some episodes were not amusing. The night superintendent had been off sick with rheumatic fever and on her return concealed from the authorities that she had developed rheumatic heart disease. So she found the lengthy round of wards at night rather exhausting and I offered, partly no doubt to enhance my ego, to carry out a night round on her behalf. When I arrived on one ward I was concerned to find the male night nurse lying unconscious on the floor with a cut head, surrounded by patients. My first thought was that he had been attacked, but it transpired that he was an epileptic who up till then had concealed his disability by retiring to a lavatory if he had a premonitory aura. He was dismissed, but went on to lead a happy and useful life as a cinema commissionaire.

During my residency at Woodend Hospital, a few of us used to walk out in the winter evenings in the black-out to the Four Mile Inn, where we became partial to a certain brand of strong ale. Medical students and junior resident doctors used to be notorious for their drinking exploits. On one particular occasion, on returning to the hospital, I stumbled over a metal catch in the road, designed to fix the big iron gates when closed.

'That'll be you, Dr Brown,' said the gate porter – so I had already acquired some kind of unsavoury reputation.

The work was fairly strenuous, involving neurological cases, psychiatry for soldiers sent down to Aberdeen from the Orkneys and Shetlands, and dermatology – a strange mixture.

I can well recall trying to reason with a depressed patient and was helping him to put on his hospital blue jacket when he suddenly dived out of an open window. Fortunately, he was only bruised, but the shock did him more good than any of the treatment previously prescribed.

Cauterising warts once weekly with an electric red-hot cautery was a procedure I carried out for the consultant dermatologist. The results were good but the treatment room smelt like a farrier's smithy at the end of the day.

During my student years I was privileged to hear visiting lecturers like the famous psychiatrist, Alfred Adler, the American Dr Sydenstricker, who was the world's greatest authority on Vitamin B, and Dr Meulengracht, whose advocacy of meat diets for patients with stomach ulcers was quite revolutionary at the time.

Practical jokes that harm no one can be quite amusing. During our maternity residence – called in Aberdeen "Howdie Digs" – one of the colleagues in my group, a strictly religious West Highlander, was fast asleep in his white coat in a chair in the doctors' sitting room. This was Dr Rhoderick McCuish who became consultant geriatrician at Bradford.

Some of us decorated his immediate environment with empty whisky bottles, girlie magazines, betting slips and so on, then one of our group, Dr Paul Heneke, from South Africa, a keen photographer, took a flash photograph, which came out rather well and was displayed on the notice board.

After graduating in 1942, I was resident in the teaching hospital for six months. One of my chiefs was the late Dr A. G. Anderson, a brilliant physician, who was appointed physician to the King in Scotland. On the day after this was announced, someone – identity unknown – put a notice on the door of his consulting room in the hospital which said briefly, 'God Save the King.'

A. G. Anderson invited another junior resident, G. I. M. Ross, and me to dinner one evening. Next day, Ross felt unwell and I informed his chief in the morning.

The chief was a chest physician who duly listened to the chest and said, 'A.G. gave you too much to drink last night.'

By the afternoon Ross was no better, so I informed A. G. Anderson who diagnosed meningitis, which was treated successfully by the then new wonder drug M. and B. 693.

After graduation I did a locum at Longside, Aberdeenshire. The previous locum had been evangelical and would read extracts from the Bible, say a prayer, and prepare to depart after visiting a patient. When the family raised the question of diagnosis and treatment, the doctor said that he would deal with such matters of lesser consequence when he next called. The principal in the practice, who was based on the neighbouring village of Mintlaw, decided to find a replacement, so I was able to go there for a week or two before being called up for military service.

I enjoyed the work and got on well with the farming folk in the north-east. Some Aberdeen graduates who were not born in the north-east of Scotland went on to successful careers where they had to speak fluent Russian or Japanese but were unable to understand the Doric.

On the whole the locum went well until, on my way to vaccinate a child, I had to drive the car through a water ford and consequently the brakes would not function properly. As I was travelling behind a car being driven cautiously by an old man wearing a flat cap, I had to slow down because the road was too narrow for passing. But – no brakes. Fortunately I bumped fairly gently into the car in front and there were no serious consequences.

After the locum, I went for a period of initial training at the Royal Army Medical Corps Depot at Becketts Park, Leeds, then had a few short postings. My first was at Fenham Barracks at Newcastle, the depot of the Northumberland Fusiliers. There I learned to play "housey-housey" (now called bingo), the only gambling game allowed in the army. On one occasion, I was asked to see an Italian prisoner of war who had bitten a British officer in the leg. Was he mad or was he bad? I could communicate only by using Latin, but managed to reach a satisfactory conclusion.

Amongst my duties was carrying out FFI (Freedom From Infection) examinations. This involved having a line of soldiers uncovering their armpits and groins so that any sign of lice infection could be noted – the treatment then was dusting the areas with DDT powder. When I was checking staff at a REME (Royal Electrical and Mechanical Engineers) unit the men were wearing zip-front overalls. As they pulled up the zip fasteners one unlucky chap caught his foreskin in the zip. He was really mortified to be immobilised in the ranks of his laughing colleagues.

Fortunately I had a syringe with local anaesthetic in the nearby MI room. The patient was profoundly grateful – more so than the Italian peasant losing a foot as he ploughed up a mine behind his plodding oxen, or the Canadian tank crewman writhing with severe burns in the Gothic line.

Then I went for a spell with an anti-tank artillery regiment firing at targets on the Belford range in Northumberland and found time to read an engrossing book called *Aequanimitas* by William Osler. Next I was posted to the 10th Medium Artillery Regiment and then went on an exercise as MO to the Inns of Court Regiment, whose armoured cars were brilliantly deployed on exercises in the North of England. Barristers make excellent officers.

About this time I had thought of becoming a trainee psychiatrist because of the year's resident experience in the mental hospital and six months as a part-time resident to Douglas MacCalman, a psychiatrist who had given me a very generous reference. Further, I had support from the adviser in psychiatry to the army, Brigadier Rees. My contact with him whilst I was resident in Aberdeen had come about following a bizarre episode.

It happened that an army unit was moved at short notice one winter's evening into Nissen huts in Aberdeenshire. Heating was by wood burning stoves in the centre of each barrack room. Now the unit was told that the very next morning, there would be an inspection by some senior officers.

So the sergeant major, seeing what he thought were tins of black paint ordered that the stoves should be black enamelled in spite of the fact that they were lit at the time. By an extraordinary mischance the drums contained mustard gas, not stove enamel.

So during the night men began to wake up coughing and complaining of sore eyes. Then the true situation was realised and we had a batch of men with mustard gas poisoning admitted.

This brought a bevy of top brass up from London post-haste, including the adviser in neurology, Brigadier Riddoch, and the adviser in psychiatry, Brigadier Rees.

My life seems to have been dotted with a series of totally unexpected meetings with eminent men, although I was never able to follow up the idea of becoming a trainee psychiatrist, because I was suddenly sent to North Africa.

NORTH AFRICA – JUNE 1943

In June 1943, an American liberty ship sailed from the Clyde in total darkness, bound for an undisclosed destination. There were a few RAMC officers on board and we took turns of duty, being allocated shared cabin accommodation – whilst the majority of troops on board were in hammocks in the holds.

The coming of daylight was accompanied by a string of instructions on the ship's tannoy such as, 'Do not throw your trash overboard as it will leave a trail visible by German reconnaissance aircraft.' Boat drills were frequent and every man who was too seasick to get up on deck had to be seen by the duty doctor. Fortunately I have never been seasick and as we crossed the Bay of Biscay we were exposed to fairly rough weather and to submarine attacks. When depth charges went off nearby, it sounded as if the ship's hull was being struck by a mighty hammer.

The standard remedy for seasickness then was Chloretone, so I stuffed both my trouser pockets full of Chloretone capsules and went to see each man too sick to go on boat drill. Of course, no sooner had the capsule been swallowed than it was vomited back – but orders had to be obeyed. I can recall one man who vomited so persistently that we had to give him intravenous fluids as we entered the Mediterranean.

By now, we were informed that our destination was Algiers. All our kit was loaded on lorries, so that we were left with only tropical shirts, shorts, socks and boots, plus a webbing belt with a .38 Smith and Wesson revolver without ammunition.

Unfortunately, my kit went to one hospital and I to another – the 99th General Hospital – at Rivet on the outskirts of Algiers. Next day however, I was sent to the

96th General Hospital at Maison Carrée, part of which was housed in a huge barn, but mostly in tents.

As a general duty medical officer, I was allocated to several wards, with malaria as the commonest condition amongst the patients. On one night each week the duty doctor was up all night and off duty next day. It was an excellent system which I later unsuccessfully advocated in England after the war.

On the 4th July, 1943, an ammunition train exploded in the nearby railway station. Standing alongside was a trainload of prisoners of war whose wagons had been wired up to prevent escapes. Casualties were heavy – I saw more than 100 myself. Because the 4th July is American Independence Day, we first thought that some American troops were setting off thunder flashes as a form of celebration, but the reality soon became apparent.

Not many days later, an ammunition ship blew up in Algiers harbour, but there were fewer casualties as she was lying offshore.

Some years ago Dr W. G. Willoughby, a former medical officer of health at Eastbourne, was a patient under my care in hospital. He was an outstanding clinician, had served in the RAMC in Macedonia and written a book about his experiences treating malaria.

Malignant tertian malaria used to be a killer. A man in a transit camp might report sick at 7.00 a.m. and have a normal temperature, but by evening be unconscious due to cerebral involvement. We were able to handle some cases by administering intravenous quinine, but not all survived.

Finding one's way to the sleeping tent in total darkness was never easy, but we had a consultant dermatologist who snored so loudly that we used him as ships in the night use a foghorn.

Then suddenly I was posted to the 6th Armoured Division in the Phillipeville area. We travelled in a long train consisting of cattle trucks pulled by a massive American steam engine, and never knew when it would stop or for how long. The coast line was single track with very occasional loops and we always had to give way to trains carrying wounded or sick and to ammunition trains.

Bowel evacuation was hazardous, as it meant sticking one's behind out of the truck door. On one occasion we stopped for several hours at an Arab village so I went to try to get melons or oranges. Just as I was completing the deal, the trains started to move off, but fortunately I managed to jump into the last truck. At the next stop I went forward to my original truck to discover that the others had shared out my kit because they thought that they would never see me again.

One of the worse aspects of the long slow journey along the coast was passing through a long tunnel in the mountains. The sulphurous smoke filled the pitch-black truck so that it was difficult to breathe, so much so that some felt that they would not survive – but we all did.

Occasionally the Arab brakemen who were perched up in small cabins above every sixth truck or so, would fall asleep, so that if the train gathered too much momentum on a downhill gradient the driver or his mate would fire revolvers at them to waken the brakemen and have the train brought under control.

Apart from our one water bottle, we were dependent on the engine driver for water. When the train stopped we would run along and beg for a jet of hot oily water and then choose to use it to make tea, or shave.

When we reached Phillipeville after several days, I was posted to a section of the 165 Field Ambulance responsible for the health of the divisional headquarters staff.

The Divisional General was Charles Keightley, the A.Q. Quintin Hoare, with others including the Hon. Reggie Sheffield. They were in "A" mess, whereas the lesser mortals like the Transport Officer, Jack Harris, the Divisional Chaplain, the Rev. George Mackenzie, later Rector of Storrington, the Catering Officer, the Camp Commandant Major Bill Writer, and a redoubtable former RSM in the days of cavalry, Capt. Frank Fone, were in "B" Mess.

I was very graciously accepted as a new boy, taught how to drive a Sherman Tank, and compelled by an order to all officers from Montgomery to learn to ride a motorcycle. I have never been on one since, possibly because I have seen so many head injuries amongst motorcyclists.

During my stay in North Africa, like so many others, I developed jaundice – infective hepatitis. The first indication that anything was amiss was that I became feverish so I drove myself to the 104 General Hospital at El Arouche. The medical pundits thought at first that I had malaria but when blood tests proved negative, I was discharged after a few days. Then shortly afterwards I started to become yellow and realised that I had had the prodromal fever of infective hepatitis.

Back to hospital again, I was put in a twenty-bedded ward, with all but two of the patients jaundiced. The condition induces a miserable feeling and cigarettes tasted like burning cardboard. Progress was monitored by the simple expedient of having every patient pass water into a clear glass beer bottle. During the morning ward round, the physician looked at the colour of the urine and discharged the patient when the dark yellow pigment had disappeared.

I was then sent to convalesce at a little coastal village near Phillipeville called Collo. There I became friendly with the Customs Officer and his wife, and used to have coffee each morning at the *Bureau des Douanes* (Customs Office).

One morning, a small child with an eye infection was brought to see me, and responded quickly to simple treatments. The mother was housekeeper to Pierre Etienne

Flandin, a former French Prime Minister, then in house arrest at Collo.

To show his appreciation of the treatment given to his housekeeper's child, he invited me for dinner. Naturally, he had a fascinating story to tell about French politics and after dinner offered me a cigar. It was from a box recently brought to him by Randolph Churchill, a gift from Winston. This I have kept amongst my souvenirs. Randolph Churchill was generally disliked and was tolerated only because of his father's reputation.

Probably because I committed no major crime, I was posted on 11th February, 1944 as Regimental Medical Officer of the 12th Regiment of Royal Horse Artillery (Honourable Artillery Company). This was a great honour and I was very conscious of my inferior status, but decided that I could only do my best.

Before long, after the division had been exercising for six months or so, we sailed from Bone to Naples. I had heard rumours that we might be going to Italy, so I had a Teach Yourself Italian book sent out from England. Each of the three batteries went out on the firing ranges in rotation, but I was required to be there every day in case of accidents, so I spent the time learning the rudiments of Italian.

ITALY – APRIL 1944

Vesuvius was erupting as the troopship containing part of the 6th Armoured Division from North Africa reached the bay of Naples at dawn on the 9th April, 1944.

Everyone on board was relieved at having crossed the Mediterranean without encountering U-boats and was profoundly impressed by the magnificent panorama of Vesuvius in eruption. We all disembarked in fine form.

Within a month of arriving in Italy, we were ordered to move up at night to concealed positions just south of Monte Cassino. Night movements with no lights gave many an understanding of the difficulties faced by the partially sighted or totally blind. The Adjutant, Captain Ongley, and I were ordered to bring up the rear of the regimental convoy. It had been arranged that a gunner should be posted at the turning-off point on Route 6 to direct each vehicle to the area assigned. On the way, a despatch rider came off his motorcycle so that I had to stop briefly to attend to his injuries which, fortunately, were relatively minor. This meant that we were some distance behind the remainder of the convoy. Now it happened that the gunner directing our regimental guns and trucks miscounted by one and departed from his post to join the unit, which was then getting dug in to slit trenches in concealed positions. In consequence, the Adjutant and I continued up Route 6, the road becoming rougher due to shell holes and there was a fair amount of shelling at the time.

Then suddenly a steel-helmeted infantryman, brandishing a rifle, shouted at us in a strong Scottish accent, 'Get back, you silly boys', or words to that effect. 'Or you'll be in the German forward positions in a hundred yards.'

So we about-turned and found our rightful rendezvous

thanks to the skill of the Adjutant as navigator in darkness.

During the ensuing few days we slept in slit trenches during the day and got up at night to wash, eat and prepare meals. It was at this time that I invented what I thought was quite an ingenious dye about which there has never been any official record. This was because the dye was made from yellow mepacrine tablets which were taken daily to suppress malaria, plus powdered army ink mixed with water, so making a green dye in which our mosquito nets were dipped, so that we were the only regiment in the Italian forces with green mosquito nets which were less visible from the air during the day.

At 2300 hours on Thursday 11th May, about 1,000 guns in the various allied formations opened up simultaneously. It was an awe-inspiring sight. The whole area was illuminated by the simultaneous gun flashes at the outset. Then each regiment started to move forward towards the Rapido River. The sappers had, with astonishing tenacity, put up four bridges, code named Heart, Diamond, Club and Spade. One of the most courageous episodes of the war about which I have never read since, was called The Anvil Chorus. Whilst the engineers were putting the metal Bailey bridges across the river, one sapper lay in a slit trench and, sticking a piece of angle iron into the ground beside him, and suspending from it another piece of angle iron, beat this with a third piece of metal so simulating the noise of bridge building and deliberately drawing the German artillery fire onto him, so that they thought they were shelling the bridge-building. Why this act of heroism has never been recorded before is difficult to understand.

Each unit was ordered to take a route, crossing the river by one of the bridges. By the time we reached the Rapido, it was daylight and the Germans had pinpointed the four targets, so the policy was for each vehicle to hold back a few hundred yards from the bridge and then accelerate to cross over as quickly as possible. When I ordered the driver of my jeep to put his foot down and get down to the river, he did so, but unfortunately the vehicle in front of us, a 15-cwt truck, capsized at the bridge, blocking our access. By a stroke of good fortune, the German gunners stopped firing for a short while, possibly to have a cup of coffee, and we pushed the truck into the river, so enabling us to cross unscathed.

So we went forward, bit by bit, and I can well recall one of the first casualties which occurred during the hours of darkness and which was as a consequence of what we call a 'premature'. That word for a gunner means the explosion of a shell shortly after it leaves the muzzle of the gun because it strikes some object like a tree branch. A self-propelled gun can move into position in the dark and the sergeant in charge of the gun may not be able to see such a thing as a tree branch fairly near to the gun. In this instance the first round struck a branch, the shell exploded and the gun sergeant had a serious abdominal wound. I was called to the gun position and was very much impressed by the difficulty of dealing with such a situation in pitch darkness, but appreciated by feeling with my hands that there was a severe abdominal wound. Fortunately, by the light of gun flashes it was possible to form some impression of his condition. I bent the knees up to relax the abdominal muscles and put on a shell dressing, later sending the man back to the field surgery unit where, thanks to the skill of the surgeon, he made a satisfactory recovery.

The next day there was a good deal of opposition from the Germans and we had to take cover in a farmhouse. So I got the driver of my white scout car, an armoured car, to pull round to the lee side of the farmhouse and I ran down to the cellar to see if it could provide some sort of cover for us. I thought I saw in front of me, after I came out of the bright sunlight, the dark floor of the cellar. In fact what had happened was that the Germans had broached large casks of red wine and I found myself up to my knees in red wine. And as we weren't able to change our clothes for some days after that, I was walking around smelling like a wine cellar. brewery,

We continued to advance. By the time we reached the town of Arezzo, I had experienced the treatment of casualties from mines – the Germans used wooden box mines buried under the surface of Route 6 and some of the few side-roads we were able to use. A jeep driver would sometimes be killed or lose a foot, so when I saw a cement factory at Arezzo I borrowed a couple of sacks of cement and put them on the floor of my jeep then saturated the sacks with water, so we felt a little more confident that we might survive a mine explosion. There was no foreman to authorise my acquisition of the sacks of concrete, nor would he be likely to have understood the writings of Piers Plowman in the fourteenth century who said, 'Need hath no law'.

No doubt others used the same device, but I thought at the time I had invented something useful. I've got notes of an episode on 22nd April when, during an all-night shelling, my regimental aid post was hit. I still have a bit of shrapnel which I found lying in the jeep, after it had struck my boot.

When we reached the Hitler Line, the Germans counter-attacked vigorously, using, amongst other weapons, multi-barrelled mortars – Nebelwerfers – which we called 'Moaning Minnies'.

In the dark I decided to dig in and, for the first time in my life, dug a slit trench in total darkness. This is technically a very difficult task, but I got into the trench, covered my head with a steel helmet and went to sleep – because of exhaustion, not the silence of the night. At first light when I awoke, my behind was sticking up above the ground – I had failed to dig a trench with an even depth.

Shortly afterward we were again obliged to take cover and I settled for a pigsty. Outside the front door was a dead German – possibly a signaller as there were quantities of signal wire lying around. When I shouted to the padre to help me to move the dead German out of the way, he advocated prudence, so saving our lives. Some signal wire was tied around the dead man's ankle and this led inside where it was attached to an inverted Teller mine. This kind of mine, like two facing soup plates was designed to detonate on pressure, and so knock out our tanks. On this particular occasion, the S.S. had inverted the two halves of the mine and attached it with signal wire to the leg of the dead German. Had we done as I suggested, and pulled the body, none of us would have survived.

The S.S. were particularly adept at booby traps – putting Schu mines on peach trees to blow off the hands of Italian children and so on. We went further north and bypassed Rome.

One summer afternoon the regimental headquarters was set up, as frequently happened, in an Italian farmhouse. The regimental commander, Col. John Barstow, whom I greatly admired, with supporting staff, wireless equipment, maps and so on, was based in the big farmhouse kitchen and, as was customary, I was allocated the cowshed for my regimental aid post. As soon as we moved into position the stalls had to be swept out by my jeep driver, medical orderly, padre and myself, so that we could lay out a couple of stretchers in each stall ready to receive casualties from the gun positions. Soon after our guns started firing in support of the 26th Armoured Brigade, a regimental officer drove at speed into the farmyard, bringing in a wounded gunner.

The padre, whose courage, support and example had always been of the highest order, stepped outside the threshold of the cowshed, so that, by his lifting the casualty from the jeep by putting his hands under the knees whilst I put my hands under his armpits, we could get the man into the building and lay him on a stretcher. It so happened that I was just over the threshold, whilst the padre was just outside, when a German 88 shell burst a few feet away.

A piece of shrapnel entered the padre's face just to the left of the nose, with a small entrance wound but a massive exit wound, tearing the right jugular, so that he fell forward on top of the casualty – bleeding very profusely. I was completely untouched by shrapnel but the blast of the exploding shell winded me, so that I was dazed and semiconscious, unable to perform my duties properly. However, I did manage to put a shell dressing over the padre's face, with my left thumb pressing it on the entrance wound and my fingers on the neck. In fact, I was physically incapable of doing more until my head cleared in a few minutes. Then I bandaged the shell dressing in position, and sent him off in a stretcher jeep to the advance dressing station. Fortunately, he survived and later sent me a card from another medical unit further down the line:

Sunday June 18, 1944

My dear Ian,

      I should like to thank you so very much for the way in which you patched me up and sent me off. I wish I could have stayed and been more help to you. Still you managed the situation wonderfully. The ambulance took me to the Lothians ADS where I saw Chrome and Col. Ph. They left your dressing just as it was and sent me back to Narni. The ride was a nightmare, the driver lost his way several times and we did not reach the MDS till 2.30 a.m. Sat. I then saw

Blanchard, but he left your dressing just as it was and sent me on to the surgical team about a mile further on where they operated on me about 10 a.m. I slept for the rest of Saturday. I have not seen the surgeon since and am feeling wonderfully comfortable.

Lockit who I was attending to when the splinter hit me is in a bed opposite me. He seems all right, tho' he says his back is sore. I don't know where the others are.

I hope you are in a quieter spot and that things go well.

Love to you all.
Yours
Padre

Had our relative positions been reversed as we crossed the threshold the outcome would probably have been less favourable.

Whilst our regiment was providing supporting firing to a regiment of the 1st Guards Brigade which was taking a village just south of the River Arno, a 15 cwt ration truck with ammunition and other supplies reached the village.

A quick-witted guards officer had spotted a fine grand piano in a deserted villa and decided to save it from further German shelling and mortaring by putting it in the back of the unloaded truck, with instructions to take the piano back to the rear echelon. The driver set off down the only possible road – Route 6 – which was supposed to be cleared of mines. Very soon he saw approaching him a jeep flying the General's pennant – in fact that of the late Field Marshal Gerald Templar – with about 50 yards behind, in a second jeep, the Provost Marshal.

The truck driver, being a guardsman and knowing that he should not carry a grand piano on his truck, was determined not to impede in the slightest way the advancing divisional commander's jeep. So he swerved on to the verge, setting off box mines which had not been cleared. The rear end of the truck took the full force of the explosion, with the result that the general's jeep was showered with pieces of the 15-cwt truck plus fragments of piano and piano wire. Fortunately the Provost Marshall was able immediately to call for help on our wireless net – using his '19' set.

The wireless code for a general was 'Big Sunray' and that for an M.O. was 'Starlight'. The 12 RHA command post was a mile or so forward, and in our farmyard kitchen we got the message, 'Big Sunray wounded at map reference XYZ'.

'Come on, doc,' said the Colonel, 'Gerald's been hit', and drove furiously with me in his jeep to the scene.

Already present was the guards' regimental medical Officer, Dr Elston Grey-Turner, and all of us started dragging the debris away from the general's jeep. He was badly shocked, covered in dust and obviously in severe pain, although he behaved in a stoical dignified way, as we all expected. After a shot of morphia was given, he was sent back down the line, and later found to have spinal fractures. Elston Grey-Turner who had been awarded the Military Cross at Cassino, later became secretary of the British Medical Association.

During the first two months, after Cassino, the regiment had 27 killed and 44 wounded.

John Cloake has written an excellent biography of Field Marshal Templar, titled *Templar – Tiger of Malaya*, in which he refers to this episode.

During this time, a very popular song was sung by the soldiers of the German, Italian and British Armies and I learned the Italian version of 'Lily Marlene'.

Another little jingle from the Italian troops went as follows:

I soldati che vanno alla guerra
Mangiano bevano e dormano in terra, fanno la vita alla
cagnesca, poco pane e acqua fresca –
a tre colpi di tamburo
tutti i soldati si alzano in piedi – 1 - 2 - 3

This means:

Soldiers who go to war eat, drink and sleep on the ground, living the life of a dog with little bread and only water to drink.
At three drum beats all the soldiers must jump to their feet – 1 - 2 - 3.

Many years later, when I made a documentary film of geriatric work in hospitals, I used as its theme 'Where have all the young ones gone?' made famous by Marlene Dietrich.

Where have the flowers gone – long time passing
Where have the young girls gone – long time passing
Where have all the young men gone – gone to soldiers everyone
When will they ever learn?

List of casualties from 12th RHA

May 1944
Sat 13	3 wounded, 3 killed
Tues 16	2 wounded, 3 killed
Wed 17	Air raid
Fri 19	Fiumarola
Mon 22	Shelling all night. Jeep and regimental aid post hit

Tues 23	5 wounded
Fri 26	to Melfa
Sun 28	Monte Grande. 1 wounded

Fiuggi – Genazzano – Serron

June
Sun 4	3 killed, 2 wounded
Sat 10	Montopoli, 3 wounded
Fri 16	2 killed, 5 wounded
Wed 21	Perugia
Sat 24	2 killed

July
Sat 1	Fontigliano
Mon 3	Messevia
Tues 4	Frosinone

PART TWO

ITALIAN CAMPAIGN – AUGUST 1944

When the Allied Forces reached the River Arno, the British First Division was assigned to take Florence. Field Marshal Kesselring had ordered that all bridges crossing the Arno were to be demolished with the sole exception of the Ponte Vecchio. Kesselring was the very able and discerning German Army Commander and considered that it would be sacrilegious to destroy the historic structure. So, houses north and south of the approaches to the bridge were blown up and our First Division based its planning on putting Bailey bridges across the river.

Sixth Armoured Division was held in reserve, just south of the Arno, and our Colonel could not bear inactivity. So we set off in a jeep on 29th August equipped with a '19' set to keep in wireless communication and climbed over the rubble on the south side of the river, crossed the Ponte Vecchio on foot, climbed over the rubble on the north side and went in to the Duomo. Whilst we were inside, German 88 shells struck the walls, but we were perfectly safe as the walls are quite thick. To this day, one can see the places on the wall where the shells had exploded.

A few of the inhabitants of Florence had remained in cellars and we bought a roulette wheel which was to cause quite a bit of trouble later. The armoured regiments quickly adopted roulette and some even had a large roulette board strapped on the rear of their Sherman tanks. Too many junior officers gambled heavily and it was not long before orders from above prohibited roulette.

By the time Florence had been taken, the winter had set in and we established an echelon at the northern suburb of Fiesole. Because of heavy rain, the road became almost impassable and there was a position of stalemate for some months. I was sent up to the hills at Firenzuola, where we lived in tents with relatively little to do. We happened to be adjacent to a large ammunition dump and were able to get almost unlimited supplies of ammunition for our .38 Smith and Wesson revolvers. After we passed some time firing at tin cans, we became reasonably proficient. How anyone can fire a revolver from horseback with one hand and attain any degree of accuracy beats me.

Supplies were brought up, sometimes in huge American Diamond-T trucks.

I shall never forget a black American driver of one of these vehicles passing a Ghurka platoon on the march and shouting, 'Say yo savages, where's yo spears?'

Then I had a temporary posting to the 17/21st Lancers at the village of Portico – a great honour for me albeit temporarily – as this armoured regiment with its Death's Head Badge was among the élite of the British Army. Vital to the success of any armoured regiment was the R.E.M.E. (Royal Electrical and Mechanical Engineers). At Portico, a recovery party went out to a point 400 yards from a German machine-gun position, and under fire, recovered two carriers and a Sherman tank. During this spell I had to treat a group of old women and children sheltering in a cellar. The Germans had thrown in a phosphorus bomb and I had to pick out with forceps pieces of phosphorus smouldering under their skin.

In mid-October I had a week's leave in Florence, followed by a temporary posting to Ravenna. I still have a piece of alabaster from a window broken by the shelling of the church of St Appolinare in Classe.

For a time I acted as MO to the 4th Hussars – Churchill's old regiment. Operational radio would be interrupted from time to time to handle top priority messages such as, 'Carry on lads – Winston.'

We were involved in the Lake Commachio crossing – at a briefing beforehand at Brigade H.Q. I can recall with absolute clarity the briefing officer saying, 'What fantastic conception is this which has reeled across the mind of our higher command?'

One remembers odd things which happened at a time when soldiers were being killed and civilians maimed by mines.

A 5th Army Group Letter Q/195 dated 11th January, 1945 said that one and a half ounces of extra bread would be issued to those employed on unusually onerous and prolonged duty beyond the passes. *died 2004 Birmingham*

From meetings with surgeons and anaesthetists of Field Surgical Units, Gourevitch and Counihan (10 FSU), Phillips and Falconer (28 FSU), Cox and Renard (35 FSU), Megan and Shenault, from Vellacott and Bamford and other FSUs, one learned how all had had to operate under most adverse conditions.

I recall Gourevitch being right up forward when an 88 shell exploded in a farmyard 100 yards away. A soldier had a torn abdominal aorta. In minutes he was transfused, put on the operating table and sewn up. He survived. By assisting the surgeon during the operation my high opinion of the FSU was greatly enhanced.

Both the late Geoffrey Estcourt, surgeon, and Mark Lester, anaesthetist, were then in Italy with an FSU, but we never met there, so that my first encounter with them was after I went to Eastbourne.

In April 1945 I was assigned as MO i/c for the operation of bridging the River Po and still have the Top Secret operation instructions.

On 1st May 1945 we learned that Hitler was dead and the following day came news of the unconditional surrender in Italy.

The Germans were then pulling out at breakneck speed. I led a convoy up the *autostrada* from Padua to Venice standing up on the seat with my head through the opening in the roof of the cabin of the 15-cwt truck.

Our Field Dressing Station was sited near Mestre and for a few weeks acted as a staging post for air evacuation.

By this time our forward units had raced up to the north of Italy with, in consequence, long lines of communication. Seriously wounded men would be brought south by ambulance to our unit, then put on Dakotas to be flown to the specialised general hospital units in Naples and Bari before being sent to the UK.

Our C.O. Major McNair at this juncture was demobilised and as I had been recommended for promotion after Cassino, I found myself, at the age of 25, the youngest Major in the RAMC, or so I was told. My next stroke of good fortune came when the unit moved to take over a 120-bed wing of the Ospedale al Mare on the Venice Lido.

This was a very fine posting, with excellent staff, dealing with minor sick from the leave centres which had been set up on the Lido, with perks like a car, (the only one on the Lido,) a launch belonging to the hospital which had no petrol until we came, and access to Venice.

One of my first excursions was to the Fenice Theatre to a performance of *Rigoletto*. Now it happened that I had been to a performance in Naples before we went up to Cassino and had kept the libretto.

When I sat next to an American top Sergeant, an exceptionally fine man, he looked at the libretto in my hand and said, 'Say, is this guy Rigoletto putting on the same act again tonight?' When the performance started, he produced a bag of candies he had got at the PX, each covered with paper which rustled loudly when removed. 'Have a candy, Sir.'

The others sitting in adjacent seats were not too pleased at the noise of rustling paper, but his intentions were good.

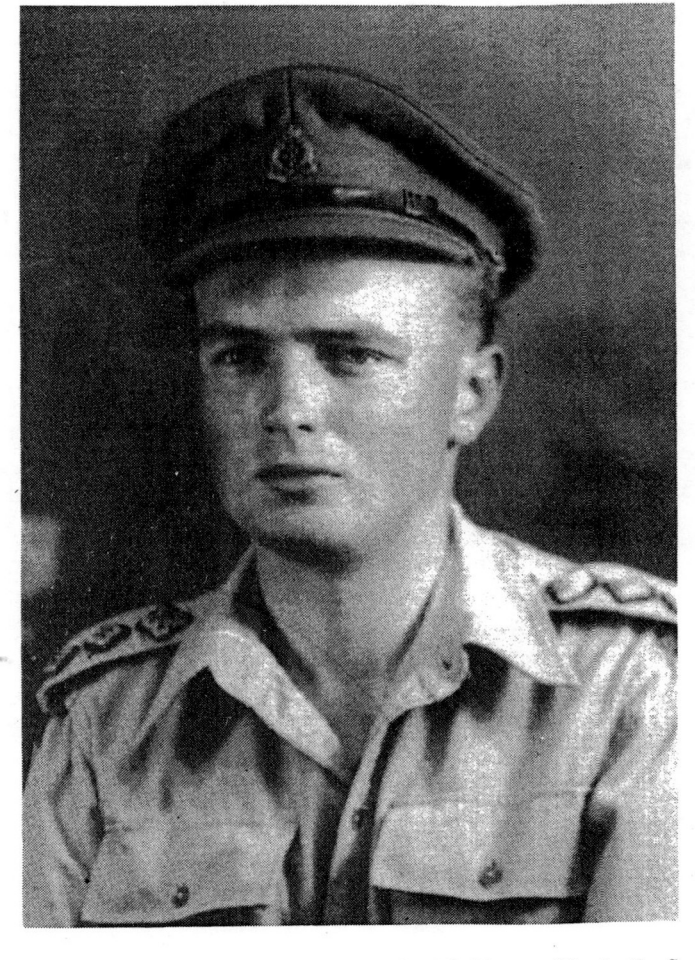

Captain Ian M Brown, our Medical Officer dealt with 71 casualties in the first two months of our battles in Italy - May to July. The casualties were 27 killed and 44 wounded, some very severely. It was his handling of these extreme cases in impossible conditions which earned him the respect of us all. In addition to these injuries, he dealt with no less than 50 cases of sickness when his understanding and friendliness were always in evidence.
In April 1945, Captain Brown was assigned as Medical Officer in charge of the operation of bridging the River Po. Having being recommended for promotion after Cassino, Captain Brown was promoted, and at the age of 25 was probably the youngest Major in the R.A.M.C.

From the book "Prepare to move" — with the 6th Armoured Division in North Africa and Italy by Frank Beckett (1994). In the Foreward, Lieut. General James Wilson says that the 6th Armoured Division had the reputation for being perh the best armoured division of the British Army and the 12th Regt. RHA as good an artiller regiment as he has known

VENICE

QUID EST MARE? REFUGIUM IN PERICULIS – ALCUIN'S CATECHISM

An account by the writer Daru of the creation of Venice on a sandbank with no facilities available, and its development into a powerful empire:

> Il n'est pas rare de voir de grandes émigrations de peuples inonder un pays, en changer la face et ouvrir pour l'histoire une ére nouvelle; mais qu'une poignée du fugitifs, jetée sur un banc de sable de quelques cents toises de largeur, y fonde un état sans territoire; qu'une nombreuse population vienne couvrir cette plage mouvanté, où il ne se trouve ni végétation, ni eau potable, ni matériaux, ni même de l'espace pour bâtir; que de l'industrie nécessaire pour subsister, et pour affermir le sol sous leurs pas, ils arrivent jusqu'à présenter aux nations modernes le premier exemple d'un gouvernement régulier, jusqu'à faire sortir d'un marais des flottes sans cesse renaissantes pour aller renverser un grand empire, et recueillir les richesses de l'Orient; qu'on voit ces fugitifs tenir la balance politique le l'Italie, dominer sur les mers, réduire toutes les nations à la condition de tributaires enfin rendre impuissants tous les efforts de l'Europe liguée contre eux: c'est là sans doute un développement de l'intelligence humaine qui mérite de'être observé.

Daru, *Histoire de la Republique de Venise*, 1821

[It is not unusual to see large groups of emigrants flooding a country, changing its countenance and opening a new era in its history; but that a handful of fugitives, thrown on a sandbank a few furlongs wide, should found a boundless territory; that a large population should come to cover this industrious beach, devoid of all vegetation, drinking water, materials or even building space; that from the ingenuity required to subsist, and to consolidate the ground beneath their feet, they should progress sufficiently to demonstrate to modern nations the first example of an organised government, and should produce from the marshland ever-increasing fleets to overthrow a large Empire, gathering the riches of the East; that these fugitives should be seen to hold the political balance in Italy, dominate its seas, reduce all nations to a state of dependance, and finally make the combined efforts of Europe useless against them: this is undoubtedly a development of human intelligence which merits close observation.

Tremblez, tremblez, bourgoys, Veniciens
Vous avez trop de tresors anciens.
Mal conquestez; tost desployer les fault.
                    Aierre Gringore *(1475–1538)*

[Look out, Venetians. You have too much ill acquired treasure. Get rid of it.
Quotations taken from *A History of Venice* by John Julius Norwich.)

Being stationed on the Lido, we had many visits from senior officers, to inspect the unit, briefly, and spend a day on the beach. It is one of the finest in Italy and we used to see men with fine wooden rakes going over the sand early each morning to remove any cigarette ends or caramel papers, leaving the surface as smooth as the top of a billiard table.

There were nearly 6,000 troops on leave on the Lido at any given time – UK 3,220, USA 1,690, S. African 417, Australian 70, Palestinian 216 and Italian 180. Each had an M.O. and I was Senior Medical Officer – Lido.

It was a busy life. One of my responsibilities was for the midget submarine unit in Venice. Originally Italian, it had been taken over by the Germans, then by the Royal Navy who had quite a small complement of men.

The Italians had developed an 'explosive boat', a launch with a very powerful Alfa-Romeo engine, and packed the bow with explosive. The pilot would direct it towards a British warship in the dark and, at the last moment, pull a lever ejecting himself and an inflatable boat overboard. The Royal Navy had put a bench seat in the bow where the explosives had been housed, and would send this launch for me on the rare occasions when medical aid was wanted. One of my patients there was Lieut. Commander Lionel Crabb (Buster Crabb) who later gained prominence when last seen diving into Portsmouth Harbour during the Bulgarian-Krushchev visit to Britain in 1956. He had been swimming around the Soviet cruiser Ordzhonikidze which brought the Soviet leaders to Britain.

The launch sped across the lagoon like an arrow – I have never before or since travelled so fast on water.

Other transport I experienced for the first time was an American airship used for sighting mines at sea.

At times I had to advise on medical problems. When a new engineering supply base depot was set up at Mestre, the local sewage system was not connected up, so a new MO just out from England was consulted by the C.O. 'Deep trench latrines' was the answer. 'How deep?' 'Oh,' said the MO vaguely trying to recall his training in the UK, 'twenty feet.'

Well, this sort of figure sounds reasonable but when I was called in I found Italian labourers sweating at the bottom of a deep hole lit by an electric bulb at the end of a piece of flex. No real harm was done, but I was able to have a quiet chat to the new doctor on the subject of mathematics.

I had responsibility for overseeing Italian medical establishments, mainly on the islands in the Venice lagoon, the *Isole de Dolore*, Islands of Sadness. Saccasessolo was for TB cases, San Clemente for male psychiatry, San Servolo for female psychiatry and La Grazia for isolation cases.

The island of Poveglia had functioned as a quarantine island since 1700 AD, the English word being developed from the Italian *quaranti giorni*, forty days, during which plague contacts had to remain before being allowed to enter Venice.

During the war, children from the Ospedale al Mare had been evacuated there for safety and we decided to 'liberate' them. So we got dressed up in full uniform on a hot summer's day, resplendent in Sam Browne belts etc, and armed ourselves with quantities of broken chocolate obtained from the NAAFI at Mestre.

When our launch approached the quayside of Poveglia, there were the children with a banner made from a toilet roll – *Viva gli Alleati* – *Viva Eisenhower* – *Viva* – *Viva*. A touching sight, especially as these children were all suffering from bone tuberculosis. I've been back several times since, first when it had been made a geriatric hospital and later when it was more or less deserted.

There were some anxious moments as well. On one occasion there was an outbreak of food-poisoning amongst the civilian staff of the leave centres, the patients being acutely ill with severe vomiting and diarrhoea. We could not take them in our hospital, so I phoned the Direttore of the Ospedale Civile in Venice who readily agreed to accept the patients.

We were accustomed to evacuate army patients with major conditions such as appendicitis to be operated on by Col. Guy Blackburn, O.C. Surgical Division, at the general hospital at Mestre by DUKW – an amphibious vehicle. So I summoned a DUKW and told the sergeant to take the patients to the civil hospital.

'This is not in my chartered waterway,' he said.

'Well, these people are very sick and need hospital treatment as a matter of urgency.'

'Right, sir, you are a Major and I'm a Sergeant. If you give an order, I must carry it out, but the responsibility is yours.'

The patients were taken safely to the civil hospital, but on the return journey, the DUKW struck a submerged post in the lagoon and sank. The lagoon is relatively shallow and no one was injured. The first indication I had of this matter was a call from the C.O. of the DUKW company saying that I was responsible, that a DUKW was worth £80,000, or some such amount, and this could be a court martial offence.

Fortunately, my C.O., the Assistant Director of Medical Services, intervened with considerable diplomacy and the sunken vessel was raised without too much difficulty by other similar craft which fortunately had no other operational responsibilities at that time.

On the whole my time on the Lido was very pleasant. I established good relations with the nuns in the main part of the hospital and was allowed to administer penicillin to some of the civilian patients with not only bone tuberculosis but also osteomyelitis. Of course, the results were good.

At that time the Americans were selling used penicillin phials with a sprinkling of paprika pepper, which looks like the original penicillin powder, to the brothels in Venice.

The time came when, after further demobilisations and

movements of units northwards, the need for the Lido establishments ceased to exist. I had met some interesting people including the famous boxer, Primo Carnera, and had got to know Venice well. When I left, the nuns gave me a beautiful hand-painted table lamp which they had received from a patient. The nuns were not allowed to keep any worldly goods.

During the six months in Venice, I had been assigned responsibility for the Russian hospital at Conegliano, near Udine. All the Russians in the Mediterranean littoral with major disabilities – amputees, blind and seriously incapacitated – were gathered up and installed in a converted school.

Sadly, there was little scope for medical treatment. The day-to-day responsibility for the management of the unit was assigned to my Stretcher Bearer Officer, Tom Nussey, a most competent and reliable man.

The plan was to repatriate the Russians and we arranged a series of meetings with Russian officers attached to Allied Force Headquarters in Caserta. It was not easy to fix meetings. They would suggest 11.00 p.m. and arrive with bottles of cognac. At that time, I could not speak a word of Russian, so we had to communicate by using an interpreter.

Finally, a date was agreed for the departure of the Russian patients. They were to go by train from Udine station. Fortunately the Russian officers agreed to my time for handing over responsibility – 10.30 a.m. We met in front of the school and saluted, shook hands, saluted again, and so on. As we did so, my staff Sergeant approached me to say that the Russians had loaded all the British army beds, and bedding, on to a truck and were about to drive off. When I remonstrated with the Russian Major he assured me that it was a complete misunderstanding and that our equipment would be off-loaded. But no sooner had this been done, than the Russians took the stuff away for the second time. But we got it back.

When the patients were loaded on to the train, they immediately jumped out of the other side and dragged themselves across the railway lines. They knew that if they were returned to Russia having been contaminated by the West, they would be shot.

My deputy at the Ospedale al Mare, Captain Arnold Blackwell, was promoted to take command of a Field Dressing Station at Padua, where were stabled a number of German horses. So we had opportunities of going out riding together, something I had never done before.

Another advantage of being stationed in Venice was that for a few packets of cigarettes it was possible to have a day's duck shooting.

My next posting was as C.O. of the Northern Italy Convalescent Depot at Lignano Sabbiadoro, about half way between Venice and Trieste. It was in a modern school and the staff consisted of our Field Dressing Station plus a Cooks' School – many of the experienced army cooks were being demobilised, so others had to be trained. There were about a couple of hundred patients.

Here, I was permitted to invite one ENSA performer each week to entertain the patients, mostly from the First Guards Brigade. When I received a list from Corps Headquarters it included a pianist, Semprini. It seemed to me that a pianist might well be popular with the patients, so Semprini duly arrived one evening with a small piano in the back of a 15-cwt truck. He gave an excellent recital and I invited him to have dinner in the mess afterwards.

About 30 years later, he was guest artist at the Eastbourne Mayoral Ball.

When I said, 'I don't expect you remember me, Signor Semprini, but you gave an excellent recital at a British Army unit in Italy in 1945.' 'Of course I do,' he replied, 'it was at Lignano and I played X and Y and Z, then you invited me for dinner.'

His memory was certainly impressive, for I gave him no prompting. He also kindly opened our hospital fête.

As by this time my knowledge of the Italian language was passable, I was given Allied Military Government (A.M.G.) responsibilities for the local area. This included road maintenance and on a few occasions offenders against military discipline liable to do so were employed on road repairs.

Although I had never had any formal training in judicial matters, I was responsible for dealing with certain minor offences and could award punishment to a limited extent. On one occasion, I found myself somewhat out of my depth.

We sent a 'liberty' truck to Trieste every evening and a fixed time was set for its departure from Trieste to return to Lignano. On one occasion, a guardsman failed to catch the returning vehicle and was brought before me by the staff sergeant next morning on a charge of being absent without leave. He claimed that the truck had departed earlier than agreed, so that he was unable to return with the rest of the party.

My information was that the truck left at the agreed time, so I ordered seven days CB (Confined to Barracks) followed by the standard phrase, 'Are you prepared to accept my award?'

Any offender had the right to refuse to accept the award of his commanding officer, and opt for court martial.

To my concealed consternation, the offender said, 'No, sir'. So I had him marched out and conferred with the staff sergeant.

'Leave it to me, sir,' and a few minutes later to my relief I was told that the offender had agreed to accept my award.

On the whole, things seemed to go reasonably well, and we had the usual visits of inspection from various senior officers. Each week I went to Trieste to a C.O.s' conference presided over by the Corps Commander, then General Harding, or his deputy.

Although there was a senior officers' club for the Allies, we found that the Russians made no attempt to discuss matters with British, American or Italian officers and we formed the impression that this was a policy decision, although admittedly there was a formidable language problem.

Some of the Russian and Yugoslav soldiers seemed to have lived a fairly primitive life. We heard of some wearing several watches on each wrist, of washing in the lavatory basin and of thumping on typewriter keys – it seemed that many had never seen or heard of typewriters. But on the whole they were well behaved – infinitely better behaved than some young British men today, who enjoy a vastly higher standard of living.

To my surprise I was informed after several months at Lignano that I was being posted as C.O. of a 'Field Hospital'. This was a completely new concept, and was named 'A' Field Hospital. It was situated at Spittal on the river Drau in Carinthia, Austria and was to be formed by converting a C.C.S. (Casualty Clearing Station). My billet was a house formerly occupied by Hitler's doctor's family, who had been evacuated from Berlin. They had left precipitately with many of their possessions strewn about the house. The items interested me – an engraved beer mug, since broken, and a military cane given to his doctor by Hitler. This I still possess, although I have had many tempting offers.

Copies of the war diary for February and March 1946, give a formal account of the conversion.

WAR DIARY

Written at Spittal, Austria during February and March 1946, the diaries recall the detailed administrative changes required to convert a Casualty Clearing Station to a Field Hospital with 150 beds, involving many hours of negotiations with higher formations, posting staff away to other units, listing and disposing of some equipment, acquiring new, and at the same period visiting Treffling Camp for displaced persons and 'Netley' Hospital which was a large German Hospital for sick and wounded. Many of the German medical staff were senior to me in rank and experience, yet escorted me round correctly and punctiliously, showing no sign of animosity.

They seemed impressed that I carried Hitler's cane and were surprised at my youthful appearance.

The military, economic, and political situation in Austria was explained with the utmost clarity by Lieutenant General McCreery, General Officer Commanding English Troops in Austria at the outset, so that we knew precisely what was happening. His account was most impressive, albeit without the Montgomery flamboyance. Another senior officer who impressed me greatly was Miss Caister, Principal Matron, during her tour of British hospitals in Austria.

As ever there were internal tensions and differences of opinion sometimes requiring prolonged diplomatic discussions. In 1946 I was far more tolerant and sympathetic than now in 2002.

So I was heavily committed to doing desk work and attending meetings. Our higher command, probably briefed by one of these keen staff officers such as I had encountered at other headquarters, decided that every soldier must learn to ski, so that we could be equipped for mountain warfare – no one seemed to have any idea who might be the foe. Not one man in a hundred had ever been on skis before, so we were obliged to treat, on average, one broken ankle each day.

There was a fair amount of administrative work, inspections, visits to displaced persons camps, to 'Netley Hospital' and to various operational conferences. However, I had to set an example by regular appearances on the ski slopes, feeling humiliated by laughing Austrian children who could make circles around all of us.

It was rather distressing to visit the D.P. (Displaced Persons) Camps. The internees were housed in Nissen huts, many felt the cold terribly, and quite a few were eminent intellectuals who had experienced a very different life before the war. It was in connection with our handling of these people that Harold Macmillan was criticised. But no one is perfect and I now feel that he was perhaps the greatest statesman of the war. He alone could curb some of Churchill's hare-brained ideas and he established good relations with the Americans, French, Italians and Greeks. He had the trust and respect of Field Marshal Alexander. When he died in December 1986, there were justifiable universal tributes to his wisdom, sound judgement, wit and equable personality. He alone of nearly all the war leaders seemed to be devoid of serious personality defects.

General Douglas MacArthur, said to be the greatest general in the Second World War, claimed that he heeded the advice of only two men, George Washington, who built the country, and Abraham Lincoln who saved it. He prized public opinion and arranged to be photographed wading up through the surf on a Pacific island which had been captured months before, wearing his cap with 'scrambled eggs' on the peak, and smoking a corncob pipe.

When the Field Hospital closed on 31st March, 1946, I took over a Field Dressing Station at Velden on the Worther See. It was housed in a converted school and we were able to swim in the Worther See or Ossiacher See in day-time and spent the evenings in the nearby Schloss Velden. I had oversight of a Red Cross Convalescent Unit at Portschach nearby and was still subject to the insistence of the higher command that we learnt about mountain warfare. When we went up the Gross Glockner to see a demonstration of evacuation of casualties by Italian Alpine troops, I was greatly impressed. Unfortunately I had not anticipated the change in temperature and was wearing summer uniform, so felt pretty chilly up in the snow-covered mountain slopes.

Then the time came for demobilisation from Klagenfurt. There was an opportunity to stay on in the army as a liaison officer with the Medical Officer of Health of Vienna, but I declined.

Our journey back by train allowed us to see something of the devastation which our bombing had caused to German cities like Cologne. Many acts of great heroism were performed by British and American bomber crews, but the policy was a disastrous failure and caused terrible hardship to innocent German children and others. It had been said that only one aircraft in five and only three bombs in 100 got within five miles of their target.

In the book *The War Lords*, edited by Field Marshal Sir Michael Carver, Martin Middlebrook is the author of the portrait of Marshal of the Air Force, Sir Arthur Harris, who was Air Officer Commanding-in-Chief of Bomber Command from February 1942 until the end of the war. He was an able and experienced fighter pilot who was awarded the Air Force Cross during the 1914–18 war.

Charles Portal, the brilliant Chief of the Air Staff, appointed Harris to the command of Bomber Command and Harris was not alone in wrongly assuming that the bombers were finding and bombing their targets. Undoubtedly Harris was initially brilliantly successful and showed that he had great powers of leadership.

The firestorm following the bombing of Dresden in February 1945 with an enormous loss of civilian life will never be forgotten. After the war, Harris was not offered another position in the RAF nor any other official occupation, although he was without question a man of the highest principles and patriotism. It is a paradox that he wanted above all to avoid the terrible loss of life which occurred in the 1914–18 war.

Some children at Cologne, obviously malnourished, begged the returning servicemen to throw them a sandwich from the train. So we returned glad to have survived and began to wonder how to resume civilian life.

POST-WAR

However distasteful it must seem to those who suffered in war, some survivors found the return to civil life less exciting than the circumstances of wartime.

Soon after coming back to the UK, I travelled from London to Aberdeen, meeting by chance Robert Boothby who was discursive and hospitable. But although he had a mercurial temperament, and was most friendly towards me, I could not visualise him as a likely member of the cabinet. He had done a great deal to represent his constituency in the north-east of Scotland and was on friendly terms with everyone in the community. He did his utmost to encourage me to make a fresh start. However, his allegiance to his own political party was not profound. He said that capitalism was man exploiting man, with socialism the same in reverse.

Aberdeen was to be more than a starting point for a career in a post-war world. In a week or so I had bought a second-hand car for £200 – a large sum of money then, at a time when new cars were very difficult to obtain – and set off for a general practice locum in Grays, Essex, to take the place of a single-handed dispensing doctor.

The work was onerous with no secretarial or nursing assistance. Patients queued on the pavement outside the house awaiting the morning and evening surgeries. My other duties involved visiting a margarine factory and a cement works.

One evening, about 10.00 p.m., a man brought his father to the surgery with urinary retention and a large distended bladder.

'This will mean admission to hospital.'

'Oh, no,' said the son, 'he just passes a tube to let the water out when this happens.' I had no idea where to find the catheters, but the son showed me the cupboard where they were kept. 'Now, I must sterilise the catheter by boiling.'

'He never does that.'

I did make an attempt at sterilisation, but failed to pass the catheter. In the end I sent the patient to the Seamen's Hospital at Greenwich. Clearly, as far as the son was concerned, I was a failure.

On the following day, I was sent for by a lady who said that her husband had collapsed in the garden and was unconscious. When I called I found that he was dead.

'What had happened and what did you do under these dreadful circumstances?'

'Well, he went down the garden to pick some brussel sprouts, and collapsed, so I just had to open a can of peas.'

A similar response came from a man who asked for help because his small boy had swallowed his fountain pen.

'I'll come at once, but what will you do meanwhile?'

'Oh, I suppose I can manage with a biro.'

During this locum I gave a great deal of thought to the future. My only postgraduate experience which might be of value was the year of administrative work in the army.

There was intense competition for postgraduate academic qualifications such as the MRCP and FRCS and my chances of success by attempting to gain such a degree were slight. The government had created 'B' posts for ex-service doctors wishing to work in hospital, suitable for those with several years of medical experience, but without higher degrees.

So I obtained a job as resident medical officer at Rye Street Hospital, Bishop's Stortford, a typical country cottage hospital with a close link to the community it served and a great feeling of loyalty and team spirit amongst the staff. It was an excellent transition from army to civil life and I enjoyed the work. Nearby lived Sir

Tresham Gilbey, of the famous gin family, the local squire, who would visit the hospital on horseback. He even kindly invited me for dinner. I was generously treated by the medical staff, who for the most part were in general practice in the area, with special interest in, for example, anaesthetics, midwifery and so on.

During my year at Bishop's Stortford, I had some anxiety about my car. A letter received from Aberdeen stated that it was the subject of an undischarged hire-purchase agreement, that the vendor had been prosecuted, and that I must either pay the difference or return the car. So I sold it at auction and a helpful patient, a Mr Norman of Norman's Motors, managed to get a car allocation so that I was able to buy an Austin Seven.

We often had discussions about the possible advent of a National Health Service and I thought that surely there would be need for medical administrators in such a service.

When an advertisement appeared for a Resident Medical Officer at St Mary's Hospital, Eastbourne, I made enquiries and discovered that the medical superintendent, Dr Herbert McAleenan, was due to retire at the advent of the NHS on 4th July, 1948. So I applied for the post and was appointed by the local authority in August, 1947.

The town clerk gave me this advice, 'Do not become involved in politics, whatever your feelings. You are a servant of the County Borough of Eastbourne and, like me, must carry out the policy of whichever party is in power.'

Many times since I have thought about these words and wished that Civil Servants in Whitehall had followed these principles.

My first year at St Mary's Hospital involved really hard work, usually 18 hours a day, with frequent disturbed nights.

Purposeful activity helped to overcome feelings of tiredness due to repeated night calls. When a local doctor telephoned to arrange the admission of a patient with acute appendicitis, no sleep was possible from 3.00 a.m. onwards. After examining the lady, I thought that she had a ruptured ectopic pregnancy, and she was becoming exsanguinated. A blood infusion was started. The duty surgeon who lived nearby was asked to deal with the case. As I was probably over-anxious, the operating theatre staff were mobilised, and I induced anaesthesia whilst awaiting the surgeon.

Twenty minutes later, when he had not arrived, it was necessary to call his home number. His wife explained that he had fallen asleep. However, he arrived soon afterwards and the patient made an uninterrupted recovery.

Local doctors seemed pleased to have one channel to arrange emergency admissions. For me this was tiring and every effort was made to delegate the responsibility. We agreed that, in cases of patients from country areas, the family doctors would arrange ambulance transport but that we would do so for cases in the county borough. At 4.00 a.m. one night, the late Dr Andy Caldwell, a much respected GP, phoned to arrange an admission. He tended to be rather discursive, giving most detailed case histories. On this occasion he was true to form. 'I opened the garden gate, walked up the path, rang the doorbell–' and so on. The clinical picture was painted in detail which was really appreciated, but he did meander – like the eponymous river in Greece, or the Cuckmere at Exceat, East Sussex.

My phone was then an extension from the St Mary's Hospital switchboard. After five or ten minutes I fell asleep. My wife then heard the switchboard operator say, 'Don't go, Dr Caldwell, I can hear him breathing.'

I had one half day off per week on a Thursday and used to go out riding from stables rather badly situated in the centre of the town. Fifty years ago, it was permissable to ride horses along the sands and I was enjoying this one winter afternoon when trouble arose.

A man, bent on self-destruction, drank a quantity of whisky, cut his throat and threw himself off Beachy Head. However, he got stuck in some bushes and was rescued by the police, who rushed him to St Mary's Hospital; all this whilst I was riding on the sands.

Incredible though it may seem now, there was no doctor available in the hospital. The switchboard operator, who knew my whereabouts, telephoned the riding stable, so that the owner chased after me by car and caught up with me at the Lifeboat Station.

After tethering my horse to a lamp-post outside the Devonshire Baths, I rang the hospital and was asked to return immediately. By galloping up Carlisle Road, I was able to get back in ten minutes. The patient was bleeding from neck wounds, but he was conscious, shouting and struggling with the police. He obviously needed immediate surgery. As there was a gaping hole in the windpipe, I phoned the ENT Surgeon, but he demurred and felt that a general surgeon should deal with the situation. After further telephonic intervention, the general surgeon arrived quickly. I gave the anaesthetic, still dressed in riding boots – this certainly could not happen in 2002 – and received most of the trilene myself as it came out of a hole in the windpipe.

Fortunately, all ended well, and the patient made an excellent mental and physical recovery.

Beachy Head was and still is a Mecca for the would-be suicide with a one-way ticket from London.

One old lady decided that she needed some Dutch courage before jumping off the edge, so she drank a small bottle of whisky which she had never before tasted and felt so much better that she gave up the idea of suicide.

On a summer evening at the bandstand, a young clarinettist in the Royal Corps of Signals band became convinced that everyone in the audience was criticising his playing. He was obviously a schizophrenic. So he decided to end his life, but proceeded to make three mistakes. Firstly, he walked westwards along the sea front and took the wrong turning so that he entered Paradise Woods. Secondly, he decided to hang himself from a tree with his belt, but the buckle broke and he fell to the ground. Thirdly, he threw himself in front of a passing car whose driver, having swerved and missed him, carried on to phone the police. Soon afterwards he was brought into hospital and after some slightly bizarre conversation with a military psychiatrist at Netley Hospital, Southampton, he was transferred there.

St Mary's Hospital was regarded by many local people as an institution rather than a hospital. The wards were designated A, B, C, and so on – the bed linen was marked with the corresponding capital letters, as was the cutlery and crockery. In an effort to alter this somewhat regimental style, I suggested calling 'A' ward Alfriston, 'B' Berwick, 'C' Cuckmere, 'D' Dicker, 'E' East Dean, etc, after local areas. As a fortunate consequence, residents of the nominated villages took an interest in the wards named after their neighbourhood. These ward names are still in use in the new District General Hospital.

Although we had many expressions of thanks from grateful patients, there were criticisms. One summer evening a lady carrying a pet dog arrived at my front door. She complained that her mother was awaiting admission to hospital and said that she would not go until a bed was promised. Efforts at pacifying her failed so that the police had to be called.

A helpful and sympathetic sergeant, on bended knee, urged her to leave the matter in my hands – but no response. A lady police officer was called and started to carry the complainant out of the house.

Meanwhile the dog darted out and took shelter under one of the police cars. Soon two police officers were searching under their cars for the errant dog.

The lady continued to struggle and, in the midst of a lengthy dissertation, explained that her late husband had been a toastmaster – 'he used to go to functions with a carnation in his bottom hole'!

The old lady was admitted to hospital as soon as possible in relation to other needy cases.

During my first few months, I became aware of the growing needs of elderly sick persons. Penicillin alone was probably the biggest single factor which extended the lives of many elderly people, but better standards of medical and nursing care added to the lifespan of large numbers. In London, the late Marjorie Warren at the West Middlesex Hospital, trained first as a nurse, then as a doctor, was the pioneer in the identification of the growing needs of patients in the chronic sick wards of poor law hospitals. In association with Lord Amulree, Dr Trevor Howell of Croydon and a few others she founded the Medical Society for the care of the elderly, now the British Geriatrics Society. I joined at the outset and started campaigning for equal standards of medical and nursing care for all, irrespective of age. Because this was an uphill struggle, it attracted a number of active, able, well-qualified young men, like Professors Ferguson Anderson, Norman Exton-Smith, John Brocklehurst, John Wedgwood, and others, who raised the standards of clinical care and made Britain lead the world in the field of geriatric medicine. The president was the late Lord Amulree who was able to arrange our council meetings in the House of Lords.

When I asked him why there were so many toilets there, he replied 'Because there were so many Liberal Peers'.

Eastbourne had a very special problem. Statistics showed that of all the county boroughs in England and Wales, it had the highest percentage of people aged 65 and over, with East Sussex the leader amongst administrative counties. Furthermore, there were major disparities in the distribution of Exchequer monies for health care. I was able to demonstrate for example that in the early days Hastings received £15 per annum per head of population to provide hospital services, whereas Eastbourne only got £10 per head. So I set to, writing papers, giving talks to local organisations like the Industrial Life Officers, Rotary, Soroptimists, Lions and like bodies, so as to influence public opinion.

Dr McAleenan, for whom I had a high regard, realised that he would not be involved in long-term planning, so passed to me the voluminous official correspondence dealing with the transfer of St Mary's Hospital to the National Health Service, due in July 1948.

Stanley Firth, medical superintendent of the Brighton General Hospital, an older and wiser man who died in 1997 aged 94, was dealing with the same problems on a large scale and gave me much sound advice. There were many meetings at the Town Hall and when the appointed day – 4th July, 1948 – arrived, the medical superintendent, the matron Miss Letheren and other senior officers retired.

I had had offers of openings in psychiatry at the nearby Hellingly Hospital and in general practice locally, but had become so involved at St Mary's that I decided to stay on, taking over the duties of the medical superintendent.

Considerable efforts were made to harmonise and unify the work of the six Eastbourne hospitals. We could envisage the benefits of a medical record system which would encompass all units and make clinical information easily transferred when patients were moved from one hospital to another. Recommendations were made to the hospital management committee that a group medical records officer be appointed. For months no funds were available, but ultimately the post was advertised.

By chance soon afterwards the annual conference of medical records officers was held in Brighton. One of the features of the new NHS was the creation of opportunities for talented administrators. At Brighton many of the most able were taking part. One was Frank Sargeant, then working at Whipps Cross Hospital, London. After speaking to his medical superintendent, I urged Sargeant to apply for the Eastbourne vacancy. We later visited some of the few hospitals with a good records system in the south of England and devised a medical record system still in use today.

A variety of administrative tasks came my way. As there were several small hospitals in the town previously functioning independently, there was an obvious need to coordinate their efforts and create a group as compared with a hospital team spirit. So I became involved in the creation of the Eastbourne Hospital Sports and Social Club, whose early history was recently published in our hospitals' gazette.

Before the National Health Service started in 1948, there was amongst the staff an appreciable sense of camaraderie and loyalty to individual hospitals in Eastbourne, but it was difficult to envisage the same attitude being developed towards a group of hospitals. In the early days as now, the multi-racial staff was made up of widely divergent personalities in different age groups, in many different occupations, with nurses forming half the total. It seemed that one way of creating a team spirit was by social activities in which all categories of staff could participate.

The club published a magazine about a variety of hospital activities, leavening the loaf with hospital humour. No comment was needed about the signpost 'St Mary's Hospital – one-way traffic only' or of the report of a nursing administrator referring to Nurse Jones who 'has been vomiting for several days and has just brought up an intermediate certificate,' and the note from a patient who explained 'When I last attended the Physiotherapy Department, I was on heat.'

After 16 years as club president, I formed a few conclusions, one being that the attitude of the Department of Health and Social Security lagged behind all other major employers such as the Coal Board, Electricity Authority and British Rail in that it did not allocate Exchequer monies to provide staff amenities.

There was a fair amount of duplication of resources amongst the hospitals so I worked out a scheme whereby certain specialities would be concentrated at one hospital and other specialities at other units. My medical colleagues were, without exception, agreeable to such a plan, although it disturbed routines which had stood the test of time. Dealing with emergency admissions on a group basis was relatively demanding but ensured that our resources were used to best advantage, at the same time simplifying the routine for doctors in general practice. At this time, doctors in some parts of the country were experiencing difficulties in having sometimes to make calls to unknown receiving doctors who were unfamiliar with local customs and geography. After the first few years it became possible to decentralise the system, but at the outset, it appeared to compare favourably with that existing elsewhere.

When the King Edward's Hospital Fund published a revised booklet on the health of nursing staff, I entered into correspondence with Dr Neville Goodman, then deputy chief medical officer of the Ministry of Health. My feeling was that all staff – not only nurses who formed less than half of the total employed – should be medically examined on entry, have annual chest X-ray examinations, blood tests, urine examinations and so on. In spite of his onerous national responsibilities, Dr Goodman found time to write in his own hand most encouraging letters, and urged his friend, the late Sir Theodore Fox, editor of *The Lancet*, to publish a brief article, headed 'Medical Care of Hospital Staff' on 19th December, 1964, based on my experience during the previous six years. So Eastbourne was the first group in Britain – and indeed in the world, to set up a basic occupational health service for staff.

When I asked a sick nurse complaining of headache, if she read much she replied, 'No'. But when I said 'What about going to the pictures?' she said 'All right, I'll be off duty at five.'

And when I asked another nurse 'What did your father die of?' she replied, 'I'm not sure, but it was nothing serious.'

When representatives of a pharmaceutical firm called to see me about using a high-pressure multi-spray gun for influenza immunisation of hospital staff, it was nearly lunchtime. I explained that I could not embark on a detailed discussion when the lunch break was imminent, so they invited me to have lunch with them in a well-known Eastbourne restaurant, sparsely occupied then as it was late autumn.

At the restaurant we were allocated a table next to one occupied by two elderly ladies, beautifully dressed, with blue-rinsed hair. The senior representative wasted no time in continuing the conversation.

'Our gun is ideal for your purpose, silent, painless and absolutely dependable. You can deal with your task efficiently and no one will realise that the gun has been fired.'

As he said these words, the two old ladies became visibly agitated and left the restaurant.

Their blue-rinse hair reminded me of one of our friends preparing to go to a symphony concert in the Congress Theatre. Just before leaving home, she decided to apply a little hair spray, but mistakenly used a black shoe polish aerosol.

During a smallpox vaccination session for nursing staff, as I applied a spot of lymph to the upper arm, the sister-in-charge said 'Hold up your arm, or it will drop off.'

During routine pre-medical questioning I asked 'Are your periods regular?'

'Yes, they go to church *every* Sunday.'

My Scottish accent is now easier to understand.

We scored another first, when, at a lecture to St John Ambulance Brigade members, I was asked how we would deal with a major disaster in our area. This led me to write a scheme based on having a medical officer sent to the site of the accident, emptying beds occupied by ambulant patients and so on. Later, the Ministry of Health issued instructions that all hospital groups should work out such a scheme.

It was not surprising that when hospitals were instructed to appoint Hospital Group Officers – Civil Defence, I was landed with this job also. We trained mobile teams, held exercises and competed with other hospital groups. As happened to me so often, I had working with me an able and experienced colleague, in this instance Col. I.C. Byrne, formerly in the Indian Army, who virtually ran the organisation single-handed. I enjoyed a spell at the Civil Defence Staff College at Sunningdale as well as a course in nuclear warfare held at the Royal Naval Hospital, Alverstoke.

At about the same time, I was made Cross-infection Officer and carried out an annual inspection of all hospital kitchens, reporting to the Hospital Management Committee. It was impossible to avoid a wry smile when I read recently that some Members of Parliament attributed shortcomings in hospital catering hygiene to crown immunity. It was obvious that their knowledge of the subject was somewhat limited.

As time passed, the benefits conferred by the National Health Service became more obvious, particularly when first-class highly trained consultants were appointed, and the standard of medical care rose steadily. As an example, I had started an obstetric flying squad, which became redundant when our first consultant obstetrician and gynaecologist was appointed. The squad had dealt with cases of bleeding due to retained placentas.

Not everyone knows that the placenta is the afterbirth. One lady sent to hospital with a retained placenta was seen initially by the doctor in the casualty department.

'Before I examine you, Mrs Jones, did you by any chance pass the placenta on the way to the hospital?'

'Well doctor, I'm sure that we must have passed a number of cinemas on the way here, but I felt too ill to notice what they were called.'

During the first few years of the National Health Service the workload grew more rapidly than the available hospital resources. In July, 1948 I used to see, examine and write records on up to 18 new patients per day, apart from attending meetings, doing half of the emergency anaesthetics and giving anaesthetics for operating lists for general surgeons, orthopaedic surgery, ENT, eyes, dental and sometimes lengthy gynaecological work.

It is difficult to believe in 2002 that one man was responsible for orthopaedics and obstetrics as well as being in general practice – the late Arthur Crook, FRCS. His immediate successor, Professor McSwiney, had been professor of obstetrics and gynaecology at Calcutta University and had come back to England primarily to arrange for the education of his only child, Brian. The boy was killed under the most tragic circumstances on the playing fields at Downside College when one of our fighter aircraft crashed. Professor McSwiney was a devout Catholic so I was left to deal with incomplete abortions, induction of labour and on which he would not handle on religious grounds. He was exceptionally kind to me.

At times he was a little critical of the scope of his predecessor, Arthur Crook. McSwiney said the only justification Crook had for doing both obstetrics and orthopaedics was that they both began with the letter O.

Gradually our resources improved, we took over a former isolation hospital for geriatric work and, most importantly, had first-class trained consultants appointed so that standards of care steadily improved.

Undoubtedly in the fifties Britain had the best health service in the world and I was proud to be labelled 'UK' when I travelled abroad. The fundamentally important principle was that patients in any part of the country had access to treatment carried out by excellent consultants, backed up by progressively better trained nurses working with trained physiotherapists, occupational therapists, radiographers, speech therapists, chiropodists and others too numerous to mention. Nowhere else in the world was such a high standard of medical care available except in centres of excellence where costs were high.

Unfortunately, but of much less importance, there was a failure to deal with the need to build new hospitals. Large sums of public money were squandered in patching up old buildings, whereas one saw fine new hospitals in the rest of the world. Admittedly the standard of patient care was usually higher here. St Mary's Hospital, Eastbourne, was in part a barracks during the Napoleonic war. My colleagues kindly allowed me to do some clinical photography which I was proud to show to doctors overseas, being at the same time ashamed of our shabby antiquated buildings.

Very often public sentiment favoured the continued existence of small highly uneconomic cottage hospitals in spite of the soaring costs of essential diagnostic facilities such as X-ray and pathology. It was obvious that only if a hospital had several hundred beds would it be justifiable to have available these expensive departments.

Rising costs of in-patient care led to the development of day hospitals. After all, most active treatment and investigation was carried out during the week and the majority of patients had no need to be in hospital at weekends or for that matter during the night. Although the Department of Health urged that day hospitals should be provided, and stressed the importance of them being sited in close proximity to diagnostic facilities, Eastbourne had a fine purpose-built geriatric day hospital built remote from the district general hospital with such facilities, in spite of our protests.

Conservatism with a small 'c' sometimes made progress difficult. For example when I asked for a pocket dictating machine in the early days, eminent businessmen on the committee accustomed to the luxury of a full-time secretary opposed my request because of the cost. I explained that my secretary should spend every minute profitably and not waste time twiddling her thumbs whilst I pored over patients' case records. Now portable dictating equipment is rightly regarded as an essential tool which saves money.

Preventive medicine includes the consideration of reducing road accidents. As the coast road from Brighton reaches Eastbourne it runs steeply downhill before arriving at a road junction near St Mary's Hospital.

After there had been several accidents there involving vehicles 'losing brakes' during the descent, I discussed the problem with the town clerk, Mr Francis Busby. He was a really exceptional person who had guided the development of the town for many years. We agreed to recommend that a lay-by with deep sand be sited near the bottom of the hill on the left-hand side.

A year or so later Ronnie Corbett was appearing at the Congress Theatre. One afternoon he told his driver that he could use the Rolls, but that he should return by early evening. The chauffeur decided to visit Brighton but, as he returned to Eastbourne, pulled off the road to have a cigarette.

Unfortunately, he went into the lay-by, where the Rolls sank into the deep sand, so that it had to be pulled out by heavy recovery vehicles. Ronnie was not too pleased.

Various episodes occurring during my stay at the Eastbourne hospitals had amusing aspects.

Whilst I was giving an anaesthetic for an orthopaedic patient who was having an operation for the pinning of a fractured neck of femur (thigh bone), the theatre technician wheeled into the operating theatre a bowl of water on a special trolley so that the surgeon could rinse his hands during the operation. Unfortunately on this particular occasion, the water was boiling hot, not tepid. When the surgeon dipped his blood-stained gloves in the bowl, he reacted strongly.

The technician, determined not to take the blame, then plunged his hands in the boiling water, gritted his teeth, and said, 'It is not at all too hot, sir, as you can see, I am able to hold my hands in the water.'

A consultant physician was called to see the wife of an elderly general practitioner at Heathfield, about 16 miles north of Eastbourne. The lady had had a coronary thrombosis and when the consultant arrived, the family doctor offered to help to carry the consultant's medical bag and electro-cardiograph which were in the boot of the car. The consultant, who was accustomed to doing this on his own, opened the boot, took out the two cases and turned away from the car, laying the cases on the ground. The family doctor put his head in the boot to see if anything further could be carried, whereupon the consultant slammed the boot shut. Unfortunately, it struck the family doctor on the head and knocked him unconscious. So the consultant had to deal with the wife who had had the heart attack and her husband lying prostrate on the ground.

Fortunately, the GP quickly regained consciousness and thereafter all went well. This is not really an amusing incident, but I could not repress a smile when I heard the story.

A dressing trolley was equipped as a resuscitation trolley at Princess Alice Hospital, Eastbourne, with a defibrillator, endotracheal intubation equipment and various medicaments likely to be required in the event of a sudden cardiac arrest. A notice saying 'RESUSCITATION TROLLEY' was prominently displayed, and the entire trolley was painted bright red. As you can imagine, the nurses soon gave it the nickname, the 'Fire Engine'.

About 3.00 a.m. a patient in one of the wards had a sudden cardiac arrest and the night sister called to the staff nurse, 'Fetch the resuscitation trolley.'

The staff nurse said to the nursing auxiliary 'Quick – get the Fire Engine.'

The auxiliary nurse ran to the night telephonist who smashed the glass panel and activated the Fire Alarm.

In a very few minutes, we had the standard turn-out for a hospital call – three fire appliances, two police cars and several ambulances, all with sirens and flashing lights.

The duty house physician, now an eminent consultant psychiatrist, was a French graduate, Dr Françoise Hutton.

Later in the morning she said to me, 'In your country, do you always take such extreme measures if a patient collapses?'

This is a true story and the hospital administrator thereafter issued a memo saying that hospital staff should invariably use the term 'resuscitation trolley' and *not* Fire Engine.

The same lady doctor was somewhat puzzled by a notice which read 'Guard dogs operating' until I explained our English idiom.

To counter these tales, she told me how, when De Gaulle urged Churchill to expedite a City loan to France, he replied in his customary Anglicised French accent, '*Mon Général, avec la vieille dame de Threadneedle Street je suis toujours impotent.*'

It was also Françoise who told me how she had striven to master our idiom and demonstrated this by telling the story of the man who claimed to have 16 wives – For better – For worse – For richer – For poorer. She had been told about the applicant for a post as announcer with RTF (*Radio Télévision Français*) who had a bad stammer.

He explained to his friends afterwards, 'I did not get the job because I was t-t-too t-t-tall.'

I tried to explain the similarity of the meaning of English words by describing how I had been asked by a GP to visit a heavy old lady who had had a stroke. The daughter explained that she found it difficult to lift the old lady because the daughter had a uterine prolapse.

'My doctor put me on the waiting list for an operation more than six months ago, but I've heard nothing yet.' Knowing that there was a very efficient gynaecological department in Eastbourne, I expressed surprise at the delay.

'I expect that my priority has dropped,' explained the patient.

We enjoyed working with staff from different countries with different religions, and learned a great deal from them. Many were highly intelligent and made stimulating companions. There were a few undesirable characters amongst them, as there were amongst members of the hospital staff from this country, and I bitterly resented being accused of being racist because I reprimanded a wrongdoer who happened to be dark-skinned.

Of course I made many mistakes – when I asked one patient, 'Are you sick (Sikh)?' he said, 'No, I'm a Muslim.'

One man travelled a long way to get a job with us.

When he said to my secretary, 'Can I see the medical

superintendent? I'm from Peru,' she said, 'I suppose you can, but I think he's insured already.'

It is not always easy to get things right when staff speak indistinctly.

On one occasion, during an out-patient clinic, the nurse came into the consulting room and said, 'Lord Blenkinsop would like to see you as soon as possible.'

So I invited him into the room to discover that he was a medical representative from the drug firm Ward Blenkinsop. He seemed quite surprised at my prompt invitation and readily agreed to wait until the end of the clinic to discuss the various products.

By simply treating everyone alike, it was possible to enhance the team spirit and benefit the patients. Fortunately I was able to put some new entrants at their ease by speaking a few words of their native language. It is not necessary to learn more than short phrases such as Welcome – We hope that you will enjoy working here. It is undesirable to ramble on too long – G.B. Shaw wrote of Brahms's *German Requiem*, 'It has made so many of us wish we were dead' – but a brief cheerful greeting is a good start.

It was part of my duty to assist in the interviewing of newly appointed young doctors – some were keen, some inarticulate, some verbose, others produced a curriculum vitae of inordinate length.

One man wrote about his early scholastic achievements, including the phrase, 'First in the egg and spoon race.' It was difficult to see how this would help him to cope with the initial treatment of acutely ill patients.

When I asked a young doctor, whose father owned a garage, why he had chosen medicine as a career he explained that he sought his father's advice. Should it be medicine or the family garage business?

'Stick to the garage,' said the father, 'you can always

back out of that,' but the lad went on to medical school and has since done extremely well. Each year the standard of applicants improves and I ceased to be involved in staff appointments many years ago.

Nursing staff were taught first-aid work, including mouth to mouth resuscitation. When an enthusiastic nursing student found a gentleman lying in the gutter she thought that he was in need of such intervention.

He reacted vigorously, saying 'I don't know what you are doing, Miss. I'm just trying to recover a coin which seems to have fallen down a grating.'

TEAM WORK

Few aspects of life at school or university involved team work. Although the army was essentially an autocratic organisation, many of us preferred the simplicity of giving orders which were obeyed, without the extensive committee deliberations which dominated our lives after demobilisation. Field Marshall Alanbrooke's diaries showed that he expected to be obeyed and was dismissive of those who held opinions at variance with his own. The autocracy of dictators such as Stalin, Hitler and Mussolini was fortunately influenced by intelligence well above the average. The world benefited from democrats like Roosevelt whose views were favourably modified by their advisers, and by the aristocratic Churchill who modelled his policies on those of Wellington, but respected the wide experience and stability of Alanbrooke.

If my own methods of working were not shaped by hero-worship it must have been in part due to the absence in 1946 of the voluminous autobiographies, biographies and diaries of the great.

Medical services at that time were under-funded so that

we were obliged to make the best use of available resources. My own dominant feelings of inadequacy led to reliance on others, fortunately mainly of my own choice. Staffing appointments were increasingly decided by committee where decisions were influenced by carefully thought out memos.

No junior medical staff were available in 1947 but the inception of the NHS in July 1948 led to a steady increase, albeit insufficient for the growing workload.

Later, it was my good fortune to have an excellent registrar, some first class senior nursing staff and outstanding secretarial help.

For example, when doing ward rounds, I dictated at the foot of the bed, using a hand held dictaphone, 'Mr XYZ is making good progress. We should repeat the chest X-ray, check the blood pressure – action by junior doctor. Has the weight increased? – ward sister or charge nurse. Let us know the response to physiotherapy and occupational therapy. Find out about the home conditions and likely support from relatives – health visitor and social workers. Probably for discharge from hospital in 10 days time.' The patient could hear what was being said, as could the ward team.

The comments were then typed on the case sheet to ensure that all day and night staff concerned were aware of our intentions.

This made my work easy – for the last ten years I never put pen to paper apart from signing letters.

All out-patient clinics were dealt with in the same way. We had initiated a dental examination for all new cases admitted. The dental surgeon with a sessional contract recorded on the patient's notes his findings and proposed treatment. Many elderly people, especially from country districts had carious teeth and seemed to improve after dental treatment.

All new patients admitted were examined by a chiropodist who recorded his findings on the case notes and his recommended treatment.

At the end of the round we sat around the table and had a discussion about the day's events.

B.M.A.

'The BMA? Isn't that the doctor's trade union? They seem to do pretty well when it comes to looking after their own interests.' This is the kind of reaction commonly held in the community. In fact the constitution of the British Medical Association says that the primary objects for which it is established are the promotion of the medical and allied sciences and the maintenance of the honour and interests of the medical profession. No word of the patient you note, but they benefit inevitably from these objectives.

On qualifying in 1942, I became a member, took a continuing interest in BMA activities but played no active part until after the war.

As an avowed medical administrator, I was nominated as the representative of the Eastbourne Division of the BMA in 1949, and attended my first Annual Representative Meeting that year in Southport. My wife and I stayed in a students' residence, adequate for our needs but far inferior to the standards of university residences today. The worldwide BMA membership now exceeds 124,000.

The local organisation is the Division, which may have several hundred members, and each Division sends a representative to the Doctors' Parliament (The Annual Representative Meeting) which is held in a different place each year and lasts for about a week.

Charles Hill – later Lord Hill of Luton – was in his last year as the Secretary of the Association. The meeting was still preoccupied with the consequences of the National Health Service started a year previously. Quite a number of the leading figures at the meeting had been involved in the negotiations leading up to the introduction of the service and there were many reminiscences of these negotiations.

Aneurin Bevan was a most remarkable man, acclaimed

on all sides as an outstanding political figure of the century, a parliamentary debater of the first order, a man of courage, personal magnetism and soaring imagination. Michael Foot wrote an excellent account of Bevan's involvement in the political scene from 1945 until 1960. His book was criticised by Lord Hill who wrote 'that Michael Foot, the polemicist, fails to recognise the profession's achievements. This stems from his transparently honest belief that Aneurin Bevan was always right and the medical profession was usually wrong.' It is surprising to read that Sir Hartley Shawcross, in what Michael Foot described as a blood-curdling cry of a well-breeched champion of the *sans-culottes*, said, 'We are the masters now.'

Bevan used to say, 'The purpose of getting power is to be able to throw it away.' He said that he did not wish to appear vulgar when he became the first man in history to attend a royal banquet at St James's Palace in a navy blue lounge suit. Sir Wilson Jameson, Chief Medical Officer of Health, said of Bevan, 'He sold himself to the Ministry within a fortnight.' Sir Guy Dain, chairman of the BMA Council said, 'He knew his subject in a very short time. He was extremely efficient.'

Late one night he called to his wife, Jennie Lee, to bring a second bulging briefcase to enable him to master his brief.

'No,' she said, 'one you may have, but taking two to bed is positively immoral.'

Amongst his other claims to fame, Lord Moran said that it was he who made the initial advance to Bevan. But I learned at Southport that Moran was known as Corkscrew Charlie – and my informant said that the song of the moment was 'Corkscrew Charlie is me name – high-powered fiddling is me game.' Lord Horder violently repudiated Lord Moran. Prejudices were aired by both Tory and Labour MPs. Factual errors were made, for example Richard Law (later Lord Coleraine) on the Tory front bench said that Bevan had had absolutely no experience of a great government department, yet Bevan had been Minister of Housing from 1945 until 1947. Mr Richard Law's gaffes in the Commons made the BMA squirm.

The Lancet wrote, 'His (Bevan's) agility and flexibility won the admiration of all beholders'. Yet such a brilliant negotiator as Dr Charles Hill went as far as to say 'The events of recent months have made it absolutely clear that the proposals mean and are intended to mean a whole-time salaried service under the state'. In 2002 we had an increasing number of consultants who wished to be employed on a whole-time salaried basis.

Michael Foot's book is not without factual errors. For example, he refers to Dr Charles Hill being a member of the BMA Council, which is incorrect. The book is also prejudiced. Foot writes, 'Many, including Bevan himself, regarded the Guillebaud Committee set up by the Conservative Minister of Health to review the present and prospective cost of the service as a partisan resort'. This is manifestly untrue. In 1974 I wrote to Michael Foot congratulating him on his masterly work, at the same time pointing out the factual errors. He replied on 8th January, 1974 promising to write more fully at a later date, but his letter has not yet arrived.

Many of Bevan's ripostes are listed. For example, when Sir Eardley Holland, President of the Royal College of Obstetricians and Gynaecologists, was introduced as being 'responsible for all women of child-bearing age now pregnant,' Bevan retorted, 'Is that a boast?'

It is true it is easy to find humour in the field of obstetrics.

A Scottish doctor was called to attend a woman in labour in a small cottage. He was greeted by the husband, who took the doctor upstairs, and a baby was successfully delivered. The husband then sat downstairs with the doctor, offering the customary dram of whisky, when there were further cries from the wife upstairs. Indeed, it was a previously unsuspected multiple pregnancy and a second child was born. Then as the doctor was saying fond farewells to the husband, yet another call for help came from the patient upstairs.

'Shall I bring a light?' said the husband.

'Na, Na,' said the doctor, 'the light must be attracting them.'

Rt Hon. Lord Hill of Luton:	Under the conservative government the death rate is going down.
Heckler:	And the birth rate is going down.
Hill:	This would not be so if you would stop at home instead of interrupting.
Lady phones switchboard of London Teaching Hospital:	I'm enquiring about cervical smears.
Switchboard operator:	I think he must be in the private wing.

During each Annual Representative Meeting, there is a presidential address, in 1949 given by Lord Cohen of Birkenhead. I sat spellbound as he delivered a brilliant oration without notes. He was appointed Professor of Medicine in Liverpool at the age of 26 and had a brain like a computer. If a medical student were to ask him a question during a ward round, he might reply, 'If you refer to *The Lancet* of the 24th July 1931 page 35 line 12 you will there be able to read an explanation of your problem.' It was said that he could memorise a complete page of a telephone directory during the lunch hour. Despite his brilliance, he made little contribution to research, nor did he introduce new theories or original ideas. This is why he has often been described as having a brain like a computer.

He once put a poser to us, modestly inviting our opinion. A patient came to his clinic suffering from epilepsy. He was an express train driver. Lord Cohen knew that this patient would be driving the train which he would be taking to London from Liverpool the following day. What should he do?

Virtually insoluble problems are exemplified by the story of the man going for an important interview for a job in the City of London. He parked his car, got out and locked the driver's door, then went round to the co-driver's door which did not have a key lock so he depressed the lock button and slammed the door shut. Unfortunately, his tie got caught in the door. What should he do?

He cannot take off his tie, he is not carrying scissors to cut it, and, in any event could hardly appear at an interview with a truncated tie. It was early morning and there was no one around to take his keys to reopen the driver's door. There does not appear to be any reasonable answer to this apparently simple problem.

Between 1949 and 1975 I attended each Annual Representative meeting in venues such as Aberdeen, Edinburgh, Glasgow, Newcastle, Manchester, Cardiff, Exeter, Torquay. At Torquay we were addressed by the Duke of Edinburgh who told the story of two cows who were looking over a fence and saw a milk van marked: PREMIER DAIRY – OUR MILK IS PASTEURISED – HOMOGENISED – TUBERCULIN TESTED – FILTERED etc. So one cow said to the other, 'Mabel – it makes me feel so inadequate.'

In 1968 the meeting was held in Eastbourne. My colleagues very generously invited me to take a second year of office as Chairman of the Eastbourne Division for the year of the meeting. To plan such an occasion takes at least a year and we set up a committee with interested local BMA members, each to deal with a special subject – Transport, Catering, Publicity, Accommodation, Finance, Ladies' Events, Sports, Overseas delegates, etc. The key figure was the London Annual Meeting organiser, Miss Barbara Middlemiss, whose tact and experience kept us from making too many mistakes.

No amount of planning could control the weather – although Eastbourne is the sun trap of the south, it rained during the week of the meeting. My wife hosted a coffee morning hoping to have the wives of representatives on the lawn overlooking the sea. But they had to huddle on the stairs instead.

The Eastbourne Congress Theatre made a very suitable meeting place. It happens to have a mobile stage which can be raised or lowered for the particular needs of operas, and one distinguished representative found the mechanism backstage. So when all the top brass at the table on the stage were conducting the affairs of the meeting and a representative at the microphone was making an impassioned address, the stage began to sink down, to the consternation of the officials and the amusement of the representatives.

Aberdeen was well represented – with the organisation Secretary, Dr Charles Dunlop, and the press secretary, Dr David Craib, as well as Dr Michael Emslie – who arranged a graduate dinner – all coming from the north-East. When the mayor had visited Australia, he asked the mayor of Adelaide if there were many Aberdonians in Australia.

'Yes, indeed', was the reply, 'but rabbits are the biggest pest.'

The Chairman of Council then was Sir Ronald Gibson, held in high esteem by everyone in the Association. He took the trouble to write a letter to Eastbourne afterwards expressing his appreciation of the arrangements. Once again, I realised that it is the great man and the busiest man who seems to be able to find time for courtesy and appreciation. The little man rarely can find time even to complain about trivialities.

Over the years I made many friends at Representative Meetings and gradually learned who talked sense and who talked nonsense. One of my own first attempts at getting policy altered was a failure and occurred in Cardiff. It so happened that, whereas the meeting was normally held in the fine City Hall, on one particular day during the week the Queen visited Cardiff so that the BMA was moved out of the City Hall for the one day only to a smaller place, the Cory Hall, now demolished, which was not fitted out with a public address system. When the Eastbourne division had met some weeks previously, one doctor proposed that we should put a motion criticising *The British Medical Journal* for being too concerned with reports of obscure diseases and not catering for the needs of the average practising doctor. My own personal feelings were different, but as a dutiful representative, I spoke to support the Eastbourne motion, as it happened, in the Cory Hall. It was difficult to get a hearing above the noise of moving chairs, uninterested representatives talking to one another and no public address system. Dr O.C. Carter Bournemouth

After I had spoken, the establishment including the chairman of the journal committee shot me down in flames.

Some speakers such as the late Dr Gorski spoke so loudly that no public address system was needed. Others mumbled or did not know how to use a microphone, whereas some talked interminably and repeatedly in spite of the efforts of the chairman.

Conditions of service and rates of pay are on the agenda every year, but the Association does discuss a wide variety of subjects affecting the health and welfare of the community. For example, one representative moved that, in the interest of safety all aircraft seats should face backwards. Does this sound sensible? Well, one sharp representative jumped to his feet to point out that such a proposal would make it very difficult for the pilot.

After I had served my apprenticeship as a representative I was elected to the Council of the BMA in 1968 to represent the interests of hospital staff in the south-east of England. My contribution was minimal but I found the meetings extremely interesting and served on various sub-committees. There was a form of 'rival' organisation called the Hospital Consultants and Specialists Association on whose staffing sub-committee I served for a couple of years – I believe that I was the only doctor to serve simultaneously on BMA and HCSA committees.

For some years I represented the Eastbourne Hospitals Medical Staff on the S.E. Thames Committee for Hospital Medical Services and was its chairman from 1973 to 1975.

In that year I was made a Fellow of the BMA (there are about 300 elected Fellows of the BMA out of 120,000 -plus members worldwide) – really a great honour, but I suppose that they hoped I would then pack it in.

Fortunately I had a happy and secure home life, but by this time I was doing little else but work, eat and sleep. Leaving Eastbourne by train before 8.00 a.m., reading up the voluminous papers during the one and a half hour journey to London, I had to be *au fait* with all the subjects under discussion. It is simply not possible to chair a meeting of very able representative consultants from a whole region including Brighton, Hastings, Folkestone, Dover, Ashford, Dartford, S.E. London and so on unless one knows the subject. Getting back to Eastbourne at 8.00

p.m. or 9.00 p.m., I would go to the office and dictate letters on my machine, go home at 10.00 p.m., sit down with a tumbler of whisky and fall asleep.

I had given up smoking ten years previously, solely to streamline my activities and not have to bother being laden down with a pipe, tobacco, lighter, cleaners, etc. The health aspect at that time did not enter into the matter. I had started smoking a pipe at the age of 16, presumably to look older and do as others did, but these factors were no longer relevant. Alcohol was also the oil in the wheels for the medical student, in the army and on social occasions. Later it became no more than a tranquilliser, but now I feel so much better without alcohol, I never wish to have any. Unfortunately, I am not so tolerant with smokers, or those who take alcohol in significant amounts.

One of my last moves whilst on the BMA Council was to become involved in setting up a Group of Medical Administrators – there were already groups for Radiologists, Opthalmologists, Public Health doctors and so on. A fellow member of the council of the Medical Superintendents' Society, the late Sandy Skene of Liverpool, also a member of the BMA Council, worked with me on this project which was launched in 1970, and I was elected its chairman until it merged with Community Medicine in 1981.

The British Medical Association has a fine record of service to the community and is not merely a doctors' trade union. Its opposition to the National Health Service was ill-advised but it now exerts a powerful influence in promoting the health of the nation.

MEDICAL ADMINISTRATION

What part should be played by a doctor in the administration of a health service? It seems logical to suggest that he be leader of a team, but that he be trained not only in medicine but also in administration. Medicine has for generations attracted intelligent men of character, but there have often been suggestions that medical administrators are failed clinicians. When I left the services, I thought that a National Health Service would need to have an element of medical administration, hence my aim to get a post as medical superintendent.

During the thirteenth international hospital congress meetings held at the UNESCO building in Paris in 1963, Professor O. P. Pedroso, Professor in Hospital Administration at the School of Public Health in the University of São Paulo, Brazil, gave a paper (presented in his absence of Mr R.A. Mickelwright) on Training Courses – Practical and Theoretical – and an Outline of the Subjects to be treated.

During the evening after I had heard the paper, I decided to make a few comments the following day and jotted down some notes on the back of an envelope.

The day started badly for me, because as I travelled on the Metro from Courbevoie, where I was staying with the mother of a French colleague, it went on fire. Fortunately, no one was harmed and I was able to get to the UNESCO building on time.

At the appropriate moment, I pressed the buzzer on my desk to indicate to the chairman that I wished to speak, and proceeded to say, 'It might be helpful if those of us from the developing countries were to take home some of the renowned French logic and apply it to our concepts of hospital administration because – certainly in Britain – much of what we do is based on tradition and has not been adapted to the rapidly changing circumstances of the present day.

'We cannot afford to waste any of the administrative talent available for hospital administration for, as Professor Chester has explained, we are all now in a highly competitive world market for such talent. We cannot afford to dissipate any of our available energy in friction, which is often due to a lack of definition of responsibility, which in each country must be established at top level.

'It appears to me irrefutable that there must be a medical professional, executive element in Health Service – including hospital – administration. This must be concerned primarily with medical, professional work and inter-professional relationships, and must be able to deal with the complexities of – for example – the medical audit system or the tissue committee to which Dr Pedroso has referred in his paper.

'In my view there is no need for this aspect of administration to conflict with business management, if the administrators are carefully selected and well trained for the responsibilities defined for them. In this connection, I would have liked to remind Professor McNerney – who yesterday defined marriage as a state of antagonistic cooperation – that marriage has also been defined by a lady whose name fortunately escapes me [Mrs Patrick Campbell], as the deep, deep peace of the double bed, after the hurly-burly of the *chaise longue*. It is imperative that we all live together in an atmosphere of mutual respect and cooperation in this world where we see such an incredible increase in scientific knowledge in every direction.

'The need for medical personnel management has been mentioned by Professor Chester, and the need or close coordination of those concerned with preventive medical care in hospital, has been stressed. We must, of course, relate the function of the hospital to medical care in the home. In the United Kingdom at present we have a trend described as reorientation towards community care, first emphasised in relation to psychiatric treatment, and now being increasingly felt in the general hospitals, where costs of comprehensive in-patient care continue to rise. Unfortunately, we find that our system of capitation payments to general medical practitioners in the community is inconsistent with the policy of reorientation towards community care, and so we see the need to review this and other correlated matters involving medical professional responsibilities.

'One of our eminent British politicians has recently told us that there are two kinds of doctors – the old ones who let people die and the brilliant young ones who kill them off. It seems to me that there are two kinds of hospital administrators – those who have been selected and trained for the job and those who have not. I personally welcome the views expressed by Professor Chester and feel they are but a development of the basic principles described by Mr Mickelwright who, with his colleagues, has done so much to enhance the status of all concerned with hospital administration.'

In the UNESCO building there are glass-fronted cubicles facing the auditorium, in each being two highly-skilled translators for a variety of different languages – Russian, Japanese, French, Italian, German and so on.

To my consternation, when I started to speak, some of the translators started tapping loudly on the glass screens of their cubicles. Surely I must have made some terrible *faux pas*.

Reassurance came from the man sitting next to me who said, 'Slow down, they cannot do simultaneous translation at the rate you are speaking.'

Forty years ago, my nervousness when speaking in public showed itself by rapid speech. So I slowed down and all was well.

In 1951, I joined the Medical Superintendents' Society, became a member of its council in 1959 and was elected President in 1969, until the Society merged with community physicians in 1972.

During my membership of the council, I served as a medical representative on the committee of the British Standards Institution, meeting in Green Street, Mayfair. The other members were equipment manufacturers, supplies officers, a nursing representative and officials from the Ministry. We would discuss, for example, a dressings trolley, its height, tubular steel construction, size of wheels and so on. Then a draft standard would be sent round the world – only Britain had a Standards Institution –and on receiving comments, would prepare the final standard, so that the item could bear the kite mark.

A history of the Society, written by the late Dr A. D. Morris makes interesting reading.

A PRECIS OF THE HISTORY OF THE MEDICAL SUPER- INTENDENTS' SOCIETY

by Dr A. D. Morris

The history of the Medical Superintendents' Society is closely associated with the history of the London Poor Law Infirmaries. London was the birthplace of the society, but it was a very different London from the London of the present day. The tranquillity of the streets in that era was marred only by the rattle of carriage wheels, the clip-clop of horses' hoofs, and perhaps the tinkle of a bicycle bell. The horseless carriage with its internal combustion engine had not yet arrived, nor had telephones, gramophones, moving pictures, electric lamps. The streets were still lit by gas light and pea-soup fogs were prevalent.

The Society originated in 1887 and informal dinners were held at one of those ornate Victorian dining rooms which were a feature of London's West End, such as the Holborn, the Trocadero, the Café Royale, Frascati, etc., all of them now demolished or used for other purposes.

The Gawthorne-Hardy Act of 1867 authorised boards of Guardians elected by ratepayers of a parish to build sick wards entirely separated from workhouses, which had formerly held both sick and destitute paupers.

At the outset, Society meetings were held monthly on Saturday afternoons, the first part being a clinical session and the second devoted to administration matters.

In the 1880 period, training schools for nurses were being established and at that time, more than 100 years ago, the society discussed staff health. Also discussed was the undesirability of using mechanical restraint in the treatment of the obstreperous cases of alleged lunacy and the legality of using 'belt and wristlets'.

On a visit to Greenwich Infirmary in 1900, members were shown a large number of 'wet cases' (incontinent cases), which were the bugbear of the chronic sick wards. They were being treated on beds with straw mattresses, and underneath were pans to receive the patient's urine. It was said that as a result of this method of treatment, the patients remained free from bedsores and were 'healthy and comfortable'.

In 1903, Edith Cavell was appointed Night Superintendent at Highgate Infirmary, 18 months later being promoted to the post of Assistant Matron at Shoreditch Infirmary. Her memorial can still be seen in the dining hall of St Leonard's Hospital, Shoreditch.

Dr Morris Munor, noted that the society had 513 ordinary members and 38 honorary members. In 1951 when I joined the society, the total membership had reached 581, but from then onwards there was a steady decline in membership. When I was appointed Assistant Secretary of the London and Home Counties Branch in 1959, there were only 253 members in the whole society.

The decline in membership was caused by several factors – retirement, transfer of members to clinical consultant appointments and increased responsibilities being transferred to hospital secretaries. The pattern in Scotland did not change to the same extent and I suggested that by offering a prize for an Essay on Medical Administration, we might stimulate more interest in England and Wales.

We continued to meet annually at the hospital where the medical superintendent was President of the Society for the current year. In 1963, our host was Dr E. V. H. Pentreath of the Pastures Hospital, Mickleover, Derby. At the usual annual dinner our guest of honour was to be the Chairman of the Regional Hospital Board, but he was unable to attend.

His charming lady deputy came in his place and before her after-dinner speech she said, 'I expect that you all recognise that I am a substitute'.

Our renowned treasurer, slightly hard of hearing, having dined well and being seated at the extreme opposite of the table said in a fairly loud stage whisper 'What was that she said she was?'

It was my turn to make a *faux pas* at the Powick Hospital, where we were the guests of the medical superintendent, Dr Spencer. The Powick Hospital was the Worcester County Mental Hospital and I had lunch with the Chairman of the Hospital Management Committee. There was a delicious cold salad and I thought it would be tactful to suggest that it would be enhanced with some Worcester Sauce. Immediately, the catering officer was summoned and admitted that they did not have any.

The society was encouraged when in 1963 the Department of Health issued a circular entitled 'Advisory Council Management Efficiency' advocating that all doctors should be given some instruction in the problems of management and administration at an appropriate stage in their training.

After being a member of Council from 1959, I was appointed President from 1969 until 1972. In 1946, a presidential badge was obtained at a cost of £25. The badge, designed by the Principal of the Birmingham School of Jewellery, is in the form of an elongated octagon with a gilt frame carrying the title of the society and the date of its formation, 1886. The background is in green enamel, the colour symbolising the virtue of hope – which we increasingly thought most appropriate. On the background is laid a silver quill with entwined caduceus, indicating the combination of administration and clinical interests of the society. The badge is now worn by the Chairman of the Hospital Staff's Conference of the British Medical Association.

One of the final acts of the society was to petition the British Medical Association to set up a special group of medical administrators, and our efforts succeeded.

Dr W. A. S. Falla, medical superintendent of Lincoln County Mental Hospital, and I gave evidence to the Hunter Working Party which reviewed the functions of Medical Administration in the Health Services, in October, 1970.

By 1972 we realised that we must merge with the special committee for Community Medicine (formerly the Public Health Committee) and used our remaining funds to commission the writing of a history of the society. No further meetings of the society were held.

People who accept nomination to committees and become chairman or president of one body or another, usually have functions to attend and speeches to make. It is generally best not to be self-deprecatory – your listeners will quickly assess your inadequacies for themselves.

In 1949, a large pharmaceutical firm, with a factory in the Eastbourne area, wanted a part-time medical advisor to replace the retiring doctor. Instead of advertising, they adopted the somewhat unusual procedure of writing to certain local consultants asking them to recommend a name of someone who might be suitable. It was my good fortune to get most votes, so I went to see the American managing director, Mr Smitskamp.

'I'm sure,' I said, 'that there must be many more suitable persons for this post.'

'Never denigrate yourself,' said Smitskamp, 'there are always plenty of people around to do that for you.'

Brevity is vital – I sat next to a colleague at a local dinner when the mayor was speaking.

He rambled on for quite a time, so I made some comment to this effect to my friend who said, 'Time – he has exhausted time and is verging on infinity.'

An after-dinner speech has been defined as being like a

herd of cattle – a point here, a point there and a lot of bull in between.

Whilst we sat through the apparently endless discourse, my friend took the opportunity of saying, 'Thank you very much for referring me to your dental colleague. He took one look at my wife and said that she should be gassed immediately.'

The speaker spouted on – as you know a spouter has been described as a big drip under extreme pressure.

In his response, a local solicitor told two brief stories. The first was about Jones, the spy. A Russian agent was instructed to make contact with a fellow-traveller in Wales. With great difficulty he eventually got to the small village where he was to have the assignment and used the password, 'The weather in the Menai Straits is bad at this time of the year'.

When he called at No. 7, the lady who answered the door merely replied, 'It's Jones the Spy you want – he lives at No. 9'.

The second dealt with a gallant knight in shining armour who could not reach the beautiful damsel in the ivory tower, because the drawbridge was up. To show his undying affection, he cut off one ear, placed it in a golden casket and gave it to his valet who swam across the moat, delivering it to the damsel in distress.

When she opened the casket she said, 'What's this 'ere?'

After-dinner stories should never be vulgar, never critical of physical defects and, if sex is mentioned, it should be in good taste.

No one is likely to take exception to the tale of the irate husband, retiring to his flat, and suspecting that a man had been visiting his wife.

'Where has that cigar butt come from?' he said angrily, then heard a plaintive voice from behind the settee say 'Havana'.

The professional comedian who has to resort to smut to raise laughs is nearly always second-rate. Of course he may be merely delivering material written by compilers of script who lack both talent and education.

It is invariably difficult for the speaker to assess the impact of a story on his captive audience.

One woman MP said 'It is good to see the Parliamentary Private Secretary laughing at a joke he has not made himself.'

A friend who was president of the Eastbourne Scottish Society told us how a castaway on a desert island was waited upon assiduously by a beautiful Polynesian girl dressed only in a grass skirt.

She brought him exotic fruit, plied him with drinks, and then said, 'Would you like to play around with me?'

A keen golfer, the castaway said, 'Don't tell me that you have a golf course here as well.'

Then the guest speaker, the Eastbourne entertainments manager, told us about a groaning incoherent semi-conscious man found on the floor of the theatre aisle.

Anxious fellow theatre-goers asked, 'Where has he come from?'

The usherette rightly said, 'From the stalls. He told us that he had just consulted his doctor who told him, "Nothing is better than Aspro". What did he mean?'

Then he went on to explain some of the problems of recruiting staff and giving references, often to seafarers who are fairly numerous in Eastbourne. One man had been particularly unsatisfactory and was asked to leave. His reference read, 'This man has served me to his entire satisfaction. If he asks for a berth, give him a wide one'.

HOLLAND

The Dutch refer to their country as the Netherlands, which means low-lying lands.

My first visit was for a meeting of those interested in the care of the elderly and I learned a great deal from pioneers such as Dr Jacob Schouten of Zonnestral Hospital near Amsterdam. Of course I took every possible opportunity to study the country as a whole. Amsterdam, with a population of more than 1,000,000, can be seen well from a canal boat. Some of the canals have wool merchants' houses on the quaysides with living accommodation on the ground floor and lofts above to contain wool. Each house has a beam protruding from which the wool could be lowered on to carts for export by barge.

These houses are now much sought after and beautifully furnished. Because the occasional car driver reverses into a canal, there is a drill recommended for those with presence of mind under such circumstances. A door window should be wound down to allow a certain amount of water to enter the vehicle before the driver attempts to escape. If he should attempt to open the car door without allowing some water to enter, the pressure of water outside may trap his arm by forcing the door to close. The fire service has a set charge for recovering vehicles immersed in the water.

It is easy to travel by train. The Franz Hals museum at Haarlem had an audio-cassette in each room to explain the niceties of the paintings to the uninitiated like myself. Nearby is the Groote Kirke, (Great Church) and there was a coffee house in the centre called Brinkmans, with great character.

Rotterdam, the world's greatest port, is a wealthy municipality and built a very fine hospital – the Dijksight – which is in the vicinity of the dykes. I was privileged to attend the opening ceremony performed graciously by Princess Beatrix. It has about 12 or 14 floors, with express lifts which enable patients, staff and materials to be moved about very efficiently.

Britain, on the whole, has failed to grasp the value of multi-storey hospitals. The relatively new Eastbourne District Hospital is built on only four levels with, consequently, lengthy corridors like the old style psychiatric hospitals. Britain too, is the only country in the world which builds hospitals in phases – a most expensive method of building involving as it does the dissolution of building services after the completion of the first phase and reassembling the entire team to start the second phase.

Near the Dijksight Hospital is the Euromast, an impressive tower with a revolving restaurant at the top giving magnificent views over the port. It is not dissimilar to our Post Office Tower – now closed to the public on account of the risk of terrorist bombs. Because I was so impressed by what I saw in Holland, I arranged for a group from the Eastbourne Medical Society to visit the Dijksight Hospital, the Euromast and the potteries at Delft in May 1967. Vermeer's *View of Delft* is now in the Hague. It was not possible in one day to visit the Rijksmuseum in Amsterdam, which had fascinated me when I first went to Holland. Everyone is familiar with Rembrandt's *Night Watch* and the Stael (Steel) Masters of the Cloth Hall.

To go to the Mauritshuis in the Hague – its official name is Gravenhaage – we had taken a tram from the seaside resort of Scheveningen where the meetings of our conference were held. We had all heard of Rembrandt's *Anatomy Lesson*, and seen it illustrated, but there is an indefinable bonus in being able to study the original. Holland is packed with interest, not only for the student of hospitals but for all art lovers, and its treasures are concentrated in fascinating easily accessible locations.

BELGIUM – MAY 1962

Julius Caesar wrote that, of all the peoples of Gaul, the Belgians were the bravest. For seven years the Celtic tribes had fought against Caesar's legions, putting up a heroic resistance.

Belgium is one of the smallest countries in Europe, with a population of 10,000,000 and a density second only to that of Holland, but in spite of being for generations the battleground of Europe and a relatively minor partner in European affairs, it provides a high standard of medical care.

My first impression gained at the Brussels airport at Zaventem was favourable, with rapid rail transport from a pre-existing line to the centre of Brussels (about nine miles). The main hospital, St Pierre, although it had a fine reputation, reminded me of some of the London teaching hospitals, being antiquated and badly sited, although modernised.

Early on the first morning I went to the Grand Place to photograph the well-known gilt town hall and colourful flower market. Later we visited a suburban hospital at Pellenberg, a relatively modern tuberculosis unit, already experiencing a progressive diminution in the number of patients. We discussed its possible use as a geriatric hospital. The Belgians were greatly interested in the British approach to the care of the elderly and although I had been interested in this subject for little more than ten years, I was able to explain the benefits of offering equal standards of medical care to patients in every age group and of training both medical and nursing staff in the basic techniques of geriatric care. The principles were elementary, but of fundamental importance.

The first ever clinical meeting on the subject of geriatric

medicine held at a BMA Annual Representative Meeting was in 1949. There I heard Dr Marjorie Warren introducing the guest speaker, a Belgian professor, whose subject was the scourge of arteriosclerosis – hardening of the arteries. Only the week before I had seen an elderly lady in Eastbourne at the request of the family doctor. The patient's son was present and when I explained that his mother's arteries were 'furring up', he said that he fully understood because he was a heating engineer.

What type of person is least likely to develop arteriosclerosis? A statistician, Dr A. N. Howard, Research Fellow at the Department of Pathology at the University of Cambridge has worked it out thus, 'The person least likely to get arteriosclerosis is a hypotensive (low blood pressure) bicycling, unemployed hypo-Beta-lipoproteinic (low blood fat) "non-smoking" hypolipaemic (low fat), underweight premenopausal female dwarf living in a crowded room on the island of Crete before 1925 and subsisting on a diet of uncoated cereals, sunflower oil and water.'

Not many of them about, I suspect.

After we had visited some of the hospitals in Brussels, we went to the university teaching hospital at Louvain, where we were greeted by the rector, a most remarkable man, fluent in several languages and most knowledgeable about all the academic disciplines including medicine. Belgium is bedevilled by having to cope with two languages – French and Flemish. The cost of printing, for example, pharmaceutical literature in both languages is formidable and even the posters on the hoardings advertised products in the two languages. One of the principles I learned in my travels was the folly of countries such as Belgium, Israel, Wales, Ireland and Scotland attempting to perpetuate native languages when the resources allocated could have been used to much greater advantage.

The coal mining centre of Charleroi had a very fine

hospital. The wards for newly-born babies had the air sterilised with ultraviolet light, but no attempt was made to protect the eyesight of the nursing staff from its ill effects. Yet I found no evidence of trouble from this source.

We were taken to the site of the battle of Waterloo, where, with the help of model soldiers and a *table d'orientation* at the Lion Mound, it is possible to imagine how the struggle took place.

The *Ziekenhuis* (hospital) at Ghent was relatively new, and when I was president of the Eastbourne Medical Society six years later, I organised a visit to the hospital again. Ghent is known as the Florence of the North and is the centre of a thriving horticultural industry. About six miles away, at Lochristi, a Begonia Festival is held every August – the begonia is the national flower of Belgium. The floodlit medieval buildings seen on a summer's evening make a magnificent panorama.

If Ghent is the Florence of the North, then Bruges is the Venice of the North. Its main hospital is not only picturesque but also highly efficient. It was therefore no surprise for me to learn about the excellent treatment given to casualties from the cross-channel ferry disaster in March 1987.

At this stage, I was taken in tow by a pharmaceutical representative who invited me on a boat trip past the old maternity hospital – the *Muiderhuis* – where he said every baby is washed with 'X', one of his firm's well-known products. There is a well-known statue in Brussels called the *Manneken Pis* – a little boy peeing. My opinion was sought as to the advisability of using a picture of the statuette to advertise diuretics – drugs given to increase urinary output. My feeling then was that such a presentation would offend the susceptibility of some prescribing doctors, but attitudes to such matters have changed and the *Manneken Pis* is now to be found in advertising material. It intrigued me to learn that this ancient city opened the College of Europe in 1949, the first university centre for European studies to be created after the Second World War. My interest in geriatric medicine made me go to see the almshouses (*Godshuizen*). The green tree-shaded quadrangle with the little old houses and the robed and coiffed *beguines* (widows) is often a subject for painters, including Sir Winston Churchill. He certainly knew where to find ideal locations for his hobby, as I had learnt in Venice.

Belgium can be visited easily and cheaply by using a Benelux Tourrail Ticket, which provides unlimited second-class rail travel for five days not only in Belgium but Holland and Luxembourg also. Within Belgium itself, a relatively small sum will provide for second-class travel for 16 days. And bicycles, naturally popular in this flat country, can be hired easily and cheaply.

Quite apart from hospital visits, memories persist of the contrast of the fascinating ancient buildings with the modern Atomium – a giant model of an atom 300 feet high built for the World Fair of 1958.

SERRE CHEVALIER – 1962

The French Alps attract not only increasing numbers of skiing enthusiasts in the winter months, but also many visitors who enjoy the superb scenery in summer. A French colleague lent us a flat in the Dauphiny Alps at Serre Chevalier near Briançon for our summer holiday, as he went there only for skiing in winter.

Our journey south took us to what must surely be one of the most beautiful German cities, Freiburg, gateway to the Black Forest. It was partly laid out by the ubiquitous French military engineer Vauban (1633–1707). A destitute orphan at the age of ten, he was brought up by the village *curé* and later joined the army. Commissioned in the engineers, he performed prodigious feats of military strategy and construction, especially from 1678 onwards. In 1703 he was made a marshal of France.

Freiburg has a fabulous Gothic cathedral and boasts the oldest inn in Europe – the Baren Inn – where the beer seems to have an antique flavour. In spite of wartime confrontations with Germans, my knowledge of the language was poor, whereas my elder daughter had learnt the rudiments at school. One can learn by experience – I noticed all the cars going in the opposite direction to mine in one particular street before I realised that *einbahnstrasse* meant a one-way street.

Going through Switzerland in torrential rain makes one realise that tourist brochures seldom illustrate this aspect of a country. For example, the fishing port of Concarneau in Brittany is very colourful, with photographs in guidebooks of the fishing boats, fishermen mending their nets, the blueness of the sea and sky – but it does not convey the smell of fish being processed.

Some war films convey the horror of mass killings and

mounds of dead, but what I had found sickening was the smell of putrefying bloated dead Germans when the intensity of the conflict made burial or incineration impossible.

The weather improved as we went south through Annecy, Aix-les-Bains and Grenoble. Then we started to climb up, past the industrial settlement of Argentiére where formerly there were silver-bearing lead mines, up to the Col du Lautaret where there are great fields of flowers (narcissi, anemones, gentians, rhododendrons and edelweiss). There is a special Alpine Garden, unique in the world, which is well worth visiting. The zone is, in spite of the flowers, somewhat austere and was used as a commando training area. It is not far to make a detour to the Col du Galibier, the highest crossing (8,386 feet) on the *Routes des Grandes Alpes*, from where there are magnificent views – and a rather elderly disdainful captive eagle.

Our flat at Serre Chevalier was a comfortable base and very near to Briançon. This is the highest town in Europe (4,550 feet). It has always been a military town, whose fortifications were rebuilt by Vauban on the orders of Louis XIV in 1692.

We left our car on the *Champ de Mers* esplanade outside the ramparts of the old town. Just as we were about to explore the centre, an elderly couple arrived by car, manoeuvered to park beside us, but unfortunately went too far and plunged into the moat. I clambered down with my first-aid kit, but, surprisingly, they were only shaken and not injured. Their escape from serious harm reminded me of the occasion when the Moderator of the Church of Scotland planned to meet the Archbishop of Canterbury and both agreed to travel alone by car and meet halfway. It was by quite an extraordinary mischance that when they did meet they collided with one another. But like the old couple in the moat at Briançon, they were shaken but unhurt.

So the Archbishop of Canterbury took a hip flask from his pocket and said to the Moderator of the Church of Scotland, 'Here – have some of this, it will steady your nerves.'

'Na, Na,' replied the Moderator. 'No' the noo. I'll wait till the police have been.'

Entering the old town of Briançon through the *Porte Pignerol*, there are extensive views and almost immediately inside the gate is the main street, the *Grande Rue*, commonly known as the *Grande Gargouille* (Great Gargoyle) with a stream running down the middle which carries away the rubbish in summer and the snow in winter.

The citadel is crowned by Bourdelle's statue of France presiding over a superb alpine panorama. The river Durance flows below, spanned in one dramatic leap by the Pont d'Asfeld, a fine bridge built 56 metres above the gorge over 200 years ago.

Even if Briançon were not the highest town in Europe, it could justifiably claim to be the most interesting, most picturesque and best-sited town. Its church of Notre Dame – another example of Vauban's work, was built between 1703 and 1718.

The Romans recognised the strategic importance of Briançon which they called Brigantium. Its motto 'Little town – great fame,' was upheld in 1815 when it was stormed by a force 20 times more numerous than the defenders, who held out until the Treaty of Paris put an end to hostilities. During the Second World War, Briançon, with its modern ring of forts, showed itself to be a key in the French alpine defences. Its commanding position made me think of Monte Cassino.

The development of nearby Serre Chevalier and Montgenevre as skiing resorts has made Briançon a winter sports' centre. The vista down the valley of the Durance stretching out southwards towards Embrun is exceptionally fine.

From time to time a helicopter can be heard in the valley of the Durance, sometimes bringing an injured climber to the excellent hospital, which has an adjacent helicopter pad.

In August, the locals perform a picturesque sword dance called the *Bacchau Ber* at the *Pont de Cerviére*.

We went swimming in the lake at nearby Embrun which I would recommend to anyone seeking a fine caravan site. Then we went down to Italy, over the Col de Montgenevre, and soon reached Turin, lying on the left bank of the River Po. In the centre stands the Palazzo Madama built on the remains of the Roman east gate. It contains a great deal of interesting sculpture, stained glass and Dutch miniatures painted about 1400. Nearby is the church of San Lorenzo built by Guarini in 1687 and the Cathedral of San Giovanni Batista, completed in 1720.

Turin is a good base for excursions into the mountains and apart from the mass of interest in the old buildings, is an important industrial city with the Fiat works, woollen and cotton mills, plus its famous factories producing vermouths (Martini and Rossi, Cinzano).

We had an unusual problem at the end of the war on account of vermouth. Before demobilisation every serviceman had to have a medical examination and we were at first puzzled by the number of cases showing sugar in the urine. Surely not diabetes. No, they had had a night out before the medical examination and drunk a fair amount of vermouth which is quite sweet. So that even by the following morning there was an appreciable amount of sugar in the urine.

From Turin eastwards toward the Adriatic was an easy journey. There was plenty of time to think about the kind of roads which existed centuries ago built by the Romans – then of the wartime dusty roads. One of the factors which enabled the Germans with their magnificent 88 guns to knock out our tanks was the inevitable dust cloud raised by a Sherman tank in the dry summer months. Day after day, at first light, the leading tank would start up and begin to move up Route 6. The crew knew the virtual inevitability of being heard and seen by the German gunners from their commanding positions in the hills. Within minutes shelling would start and very often the leading tank would be knocked out, by shelling or mines. We all knew what was likely to happen and had the highest admiration for those in the leading tank. What a difference to be bowling along an *autostrada* on a hot summer day. How many of the young people in 2002 give a thought for these tank crews whose way of life was so very different 60 years ago.

A brief visit to Sirmione on Lake Garda makes a welcome break in the journey. A narrow tongue of earth ending in a rocky peninsula juts out into the centre of a moraine which blocked the waters of the quaternary glacier and formed Lake Garda. Sirmione grew up at the base of this promontory. Its old houses surrounded the crenellated shape of the Castle of the Scaligers. It seems to be a favourite venue for Germans and I was identified as being German possibly because I was then fair-haired and fair-skinned.

Venice had not changed, nor had Ravenna, although there were many new buildings and fine roads. A visit to Florence revived past memories. At Pisa I persuaded the children to stand beside the tower and lean sideways, whilst I took a photograph which made the rest of the environment appear to be on an incline. Then on to the Mediterranean, with a break at Lido di Camaiore, which had been at the western end of the winter line in 1944–45. The world famous marble quarries at Carrara are only a few kilometres northwards. Michaelangelo used to go there to choose the blocks from which he carved his masterpieces. From there we returned home through Allessandria and onwards into France then back home.

Imbalance was a word I used when writing about the relatively high percentage of elderly people in Eastbourne. After I realised that I had not seen this word in print the letters editor of The Sunday Times said, 'You would certainly seem to have a case for its inclusion in the Oxford Dictionary'. The word had been included in Chambers 20th Century Dictionary and the Reader's Digest Great Encyclopaedia Dictionary, the latter describing imbalance as a disturbance of mental or bodily equilibrium – used in psychology and pathology.

It was satisfying to bring the word to the attention of the Oxford Dictionary and to see it being widely used during the past fifty years.

In 1971, the journal *Modern Geriatrics* published an article on 'The Large Scale Movement of Elderly People to South Coast Resorts – Social and Medical Problems.' Immediately the article was written, I regretted having used the word 'problems'. Old people in need present a challenge, not a problem. Younger members of the community often fail to realise that the fabric of the society in which they live was created by their forebears, who had a very much tougher life than young people accept often without question in 2002.

It was possible to demonstrate by graphs and diagrams how, in Eastbourne, the percentage of pensionable people had risen from five to 30 since the beginning of the century. Our studies showed that four fifths of Eastbourne hospital patients were 'immigrants', only one fifth having been born locally. Of the 'immigrants', about half had come from London.

We pointed out that our hospital service had not expanded sufficiently because hospital revenue allocations tended to be based on demand rather than need.

We wanted a fair share of the national cake, albeit at the expense of other over-funded places, especially London, and now the objective has been achieved.

DENMARK – 1963

When it was agreed that there would be a European Geriatric Meeting in Denmark in 1963, I was fortunately able to get in touch with a Danish anaesthetist, who lived at Holte, on the outskirts of Copenhagen, and fix a house exchange.

We travelled by car to Harwich, crossed over to Esberg and arrived in the evening after dark. My secretary, Mrs Mary Andersen, was married to a Dane, spoke fluent Danish, and gave me masses of useful advice. When I asked about communicating with Danes, she told me that practically everyone in Denmark could speak English. Unfortunately I found that this was not the case, and presumably it was the tiny minority of non-English speaking Danes whose advice I sought when looking for Holte.

However, when we arrived, there was a marvellous welcome awaiting: the neighbours had made tea!

Each morning I set off for the meetings in the Technical University in Øster Voldgade. There was a six-lane highway from Holte into Copenhagen, and it was obvious that 99.9% of the motorists did this journey each morning.

As the late Ernest Marples recounted when he got in th wrong traffic lane in Los Angeles, 'I objected, not to what the critical driver said about me, but the implied insult to my parents.'

The Danish businessmen going into the city were obviously fluent English speakers and recognised my GB plates.

The Danes were very interested in our approach to the care of the elderly and we learned a great deal from them. We had much in common. When Nelson offered an armistice after the Battle of the Baltic in 1801 he referred to 'the brothers of Englishmen, the Danes.'

We were taken not only to modern hospitals such as the Glostrup but also to the old people's complex *Den Gamle By*. This has a heavy concentration of elderly persons in varying degrees of dependency – in sheltered homes, nursing homes and hospital wards.

It may be better to spread such facilities more in any community. We also visited an excellent home for the elderly at Gentofte, in the northern part of Copenhagen. The Danes were very hospitable, and gave us a magnificent reception in the Town Hall, finely situated in the spacious Raadhuspladsen (Town Hall Square). From the square leads the Bond Street of Copenhagen, the Strøget. Most visitors want to see what many regard as the symbol of Copenhagen, *Den Lille Havefrue* (the Little Mermaid), overlooking the harbour. The New Harbour (*Nyhavn*) has acquired a rather bad reputation and is best avoided by anyone who wants to keep out of trouble.

Southend is to London what Klampenberg used to be for Copenhagen, but is now avoided by beach lovers on account of sewage effluent. There are fine beaches on the north coast at Hornbaek and Hillebaek, and if you have cultural interests, Elsinore is quite near. Incidentally, there is a jetfoil service over to Sweden which is inexpensive and takes only 25 minutes.

The original royal palace, Christiansborg, is in the north, but the King and Queen live in Amalienborg Palace in Copenhagen. By mistake I drove into the courtyard one evening but was courteously and firmly ejected in a few moments.

Shortage of time prevented us from seeing many innumerable fascinating aspects of Denmark. Some were modern and known worldwide – the Carlsberg and Tuborg breweries – spotlessly clean and full of stainless steel brewing equipment. Rightly, only modest samples are available at the end of the tour. Just as in the Guinness Brewery in Dublin, one has to walk for miles before tasting a small mug of the famous brew. Therefore in Denmark there is no encouragement to visit the breweries merely to obtain a free sample.

The suburban electric S-train (*S-Tog*) is much used by Copenhageners. Sometimes I took the *S-Tog* from Holte to meetings in the Technical University.

We managed to fit in a visit to Frederiksborg Castle at Hillerod with its fine museum administered by the Carlsberg Foundation. I took a photograph of the Knights' Hall, containing furniture from the time of Christian IV – seventeenth century.

At nearby Trelleborg, a vast Viking military camp was excavated between 1934–1941. It has been estimated that it was constructed in 990–1000 AD. Historians can visit Bromme where the earliest traces of human habitation in Denmark were discovered, dating from 8,000 to 10,000 BC.

Hans Christian Andersen must be the favourite storyteller of millions and his house is in the town of Odense on Jutland. It is now a museum, with leather-covered walls, Bornholm tiles, beautiful hand-woven carpets, marble from Sicily, Carrara, and Belgium, with non-slip stone from Norway on the floors.

Like so many highly intelligent famous men, Hans Christian Andresen had abnormal traits of personality. He feared that he would be trapped in a burning building, so carried with him on his lecture tours of the United States a coil of rope with which he could lower himself to the ground from the bedroom of his burning hotel. This coil of rope is on display in the museum, along with his top hat in a leather case.

Not far away in Roskilde which, in its early days, was the most important city in Denmark, being the seat of the Danish Kings from 1020 until 1416.

It has a magnificent cathedral – the Roskilde *Domkirke*.

Where it differed from the many other cathedrals visited, other than Strasbourg, was that it had an extraordinary clock. Mechanical figures strike the hours and quarters. There is an effigy of St George whose horse rears up with the stroke of every hour and a dragon that as regularly lets out a piercing squeal. Nearby, after the cultural feast, it is possible to work off surplus energy in a fine swimming pool built at the base of a water tower.

Swimming in the sea is very refreshing at Hornbaek on the north coast of Zealand, with superb beaches. Back in Copenhagen, the world-famous Tivoli gardens provide every conceivable form of outdoor entertainment.

Memories of Denmark, both from studies of its health services and from tourist visits, persist undimmed.

ISRAEL – NOVEMBER 1964

There appeared to be similarities between two relatively small countries – Israel and Finland. Both had overcome adversity, both had proud nationals, pleased to extol the virtues of their native land, and both had languages which were difficult to learn. 'Shalom' is the customary Israeli greeting.

In November 1964, as a member of the International Hospital Federation, I spent two weeks in Israel studying its health services, representing the British Medical Association to whom I reported on my return. My companion was the late Dr Ian Murray Macgregor of Edinburgh, then a Principal Medical Officer at the Scottish Home and Health Department. He was a distinguished graduate of Edinburgh University and the son of a famous Medical Officer of Health for Glasgow. No one could have been a more interesting and delightful colleague and we shared a room at the Dan Hotel in Tel Aviv.

The flight from London takes about four and a half hours and we went directly from Lod Airport at Tel Aviv to our hotel. Before dinner, we went down to the bar on the ground floor and here found Moshe Dyan extolling the virtues of the Israeli army to a group of journalists, fortunately for us speaking in English.

He was Chief of State at the time of the Sinai Campaign, Minister of Defence during the Six Day War, and later the Yom Kippur War. Dayan is the Russian word for judge and his father was a judge in Kiev before going to Israel. As a child he was in a kibbutz in Daganiah, joined the Haganah – the underground Jewish self-defence organisation – at the age of 16 and was imprisoned in Acre for 15 months. Nevertheless he helped the British Army in Syria during the Second World War and lost an eye in combat.

He was a protegé of Ben Gurion and in his autobiography he tells of his early struggles, his conflict with the views of some of his own countrymen and his fascinating experiences.

Many of the Israeli hospitals are run by the trade union organisation the Histadrut and we started by visiting the main hospital in Tel Aviv. It was staffed by Jews of various nationalities providing excellent standards of care but was very crowded, with beds in the corridors because the population of Israel was increasing so rapidly. I took a number of photographs of the wards, their equipment and the patients.

Nearby was the Tel Hashomer Hospital, a hutted building, described as being a beautiful watch in a rough casing.

The city of Tel Aviv is of modern concrete construction, many of the houses having solar heaters which provide all the hot water required. Although our visit was in November the weather was fine and we experienced the *khamsin*, or desert wind, warmer than the *mistral* in France but not dissimilar to the trade winds of the West Indies. It was possible to get around in Tel Aviv by taxi – a *sharut* – which can take up to seven passengers and costs much the same as public transport. The currency is the shekel divided into ten liras (Hebrew – *lirot*).

Saturday is the Jewish sabbath, and we enjoyed the local diet of *gefülte* fish, chopped liver, chicken soup and Israeli yoghourt called *labin*.

It helps to learn a brief glossary of terms when visiting different areas. *Ein* means fountain, *beth*, a house, *beer*, a well, *rehov*, a street, *souk*, a market and *wadi*, a river bed.

Israel was proclaimed an independent state on 14th May, 1948, the Balfour Declaration of 1917 having asserted that a Jewish National Home should be established by Israel.

Government of the 4,000,000 inhabitants is by the parliament, called the Knesset, with 120 members. Here one can see a huge sculptured *menorah* or seven-branched candelabrum. The population consists of about 3.5 million Jews, 400,000 Moslems, 80,000 Christians and 44,000 Druze, Bahai, etc.

Jerusalem was proclaimed capital of Israel in 1950. It has a population of about 360,000 and some of the interesting parts we saw were the Khan – a restored Turkish caravanserai for travellers who in earlier times reached Jerusalem after the city gates were closed for the night. Being a Scot, I was naturally interested in St Andrew's Scottish Church and Hospice. Visitors usually visit the Jaffa Gate and Dome of the Rock.

Many of the world's leading artists – Pablo Casals, Isaac Stern, Arthur Rubenstein, Saul Bellow, Yehudi Menuhin and numerous other distinguished figures have enjoyed coming to Israel to share their talents with visitors and local residents.

The Israel Museum is fascinating, containing the Dead Sea Scrolls, found in 1947. It is in a complex of buildings, including the Hebrew University, National Library, University Stadium, Planetarium, Wise Auditorium and Synagogue. Also there is an eighteenth-century synagogue from Vittorio Veneto, a small town near Venice.

We must never forget that 6,000,000 Jews were killed by the Nazis, so that the names of Auschwitz, Bergen-Belsen, Buchenwald, Dachau and many others are deeply engraved in the memory.

Nearby is Gethsemane, said to be so called from the name of a shallow cave used by Israelite farmers thousands of years ago to prepare olive oil. The Hebrew word for an olive oil press is *gat shemen*.

Ein Karem, the birthplace of John the Baptist, is now the site of the Hadassah Medical Centre. It is a very fine building, designed like the segments of an orange, with the critically-ill patients near the centre and ward day rooms on the outer aspect. I talked to a number of patients including a charming old lady in a single room.

'I hope,' I said, 'that you are getting good treatment here.'

'I believe so,' she replied and explained that her husband was the Professor of Surgery.

She kindly allowed me to take her photograph. We then visited the hospital chapel, or rather the synagogue, having to put on black skull caps before going in. Here are the famous stained-glass windows by Chagall.

I felt that the hospital was a little too far from the city of Jerusalem as it made attendances by outpatients somewhat difficult.

Whilst having lunch at the hospital canteen, I spoke to the chief pharmacist who came from the United States and was earning a much smaller salary in Israel. But he said it was worth it to ensure that his family grew up there.

As in Holland, visits to various parts of Israel are easy because it is relatively small (8,000 sq. miles) being only 260 miles from north to south and between 12 and 72 miles at various points from east to west.

Jericho is easily accessible. It is one of the oldest cities in the world – a tower dating from 8,000 BC has been excavated.

The Sea of Galilee is below sea level and concrete aqueducts have been built around the periphery to take away the salt water. From Galilee, water is pumped through large pipes made of concrete segments, carrying water to irrigate the land with branches leading off the main aqueduct like the branches of a tree. At the end of each 'twig' is a sprinkler, some of which I photographed. It is really quite remarkable to see the difference between the lush vegetation of the irrigated areas growing citrus fruits, vegetables and so on, and the non-irrigated areas. We visited Tiberias (population 35,000) and Nazareth (population 40,000) – it is one of the largest Arab centres in Israel.

Going south from Jerusalem, Bethlehem is about six miles distant. The name means 'House of Bread' and the people living there are mostly Christian Arabs.

Beersheba (or Be'er Sheva) is further south and we spent some time in the Central Hospital there. Not only Jews but also Bedouins receive treatment in this hospital. Even then, the Israeli architects had planned the building on the assumption that there might be a war and that there would be no electricity supply. So there were ramps leading up to each floor which must have been a very costly addition to the building.

We were taken to a Bedouin encampment and offered small cups of thick sugary black coffee. Camel rides were available, but I declined because it was obvious that the camels were all flea-ridden. Whilst some of my colleagues sampled camel transport I took photographs, one, of a camel's head silhouetted against the setting sun, coming out well.

Masada (Hebrew – *metsada* or *metsuda* meaning a stronghold) is a flat-topped mass of rock, 1,300 feet. above the shore of the Dead Sea. When the Romans took Masada in AD 73, the 960 Jewish defendants killed themselves rather than be captured, leaving stores of food to show that they chose death rather than slavery.

Most visitors go to Eilat on the Red Sea for water sports and visit King Solomon's Mines about eight miles away, but we missed this and went instead to Ashkelon, 35 miles south of Tel Aviv. Not many people know that *caepa ascalonia* cultivated there by the Romans is what the French called *échalote*, or the English shallots. Nearby is a deep-water port called Ashdod built by Israel, with a massive breakwater made from huge blocks of stone and concrete.

On the way back to Tel Aviv, we stopped for a time at Jaffa, named after Japhet, son of Noah. It is no longer an important harbour, but is a picturesque town where artists and craftsmen choose to live. We were told that Jaffa oranges should now really be called Haifa oranges.

No visit to Tel Aviv is complete without seeing the Weizman Institute, named after Chaim Weizman, who lived at nearby Rehovat from 1934. He was a Jewish research chemist from Manchester who became the First President of Israel. At the institute is a water desalination plant.

Caesarea, just a few miles north of Tel Aviv, was founded by Herod in the first century BC and has a magnificent open-air amphitheatre which makes an excellent venue for celebrity concerts.

Then on to Mount Carmel, from which there is a fine view over the bay to Acre, somewhat reminiscent of the Bay of Naples. The Ram Bam hospital in Haifa provides an excellent standard of medical care. One of the prominent landmarks is the Bahai Temple, with its gilt cupola. The Bahai Faith, said to encompass all faiths, originated in Iran in the nineteenth century.

A visit to Acre is well worthwhile. There glass was discovered and it now has an interesting market. When we entered the mosque we had to go barefoot. The call to prayer was coming from a loudspeaker at the top, the switch being operated by a somewhat languid Arab at the front door.

The general impact gained was of a proud country, where the local inhabitants, who call themselves *sabra* i.e. cactus, are intensely interested in the history of their country, advise the visitor to use the Bible as a guidebook and provide an excellent medical service which compared favourably with that in other countries visited.

SWEDEN – JUNE 1965

The fact that Sweden is a wealthy and prosperous country is not obvious in an ostentatious way, but at the time of my visit, the hospitals seemed to be staffed and equipped to a higher standard than in most other countries. The population is about twice as great as that of Norway, totalling now nearly nine millions.

Everyone has heard of Swedish iron ore and Swedish steel.

Strindberg is acknowledged as a genius on the brink of madness who produced a constant flow of brilliant books and plays known the world over. That I consider him to be a psychopath is no doubt evidence of my own abnormal outlook.

Another name recognised throughout the world is Nobel. It seems paradoxical that Alfred Nobel should have become enormously wealthy through explosives yet be remembered for his peace prize. He never settled anywhere, was described by Eric Elstob in his excellent book on Sweden as the richest tramp in Europe, and never married. He died in 1896. Although he had made his fortune from dynamite, he was an active pacifist. He said, 'My factories will end war sooner than your conferences.' He meant that they would do so by making the weapons of war too destructive.

This concept is even more true today. No rational person wants to commit suicide and the world knows that a nuclear war would be the end of our civilisation.

Sweden and Switzerland are probably the most prosperous countries in the world. The Karolinska Hospital is world-famous for its high standards and original research work. In the field of geriatric medicine, I recall being impressed by the hospital at Blackberg, on the outskirts of

Stockholm, where there was a happy atmosphere in a beautifully equipped and well-staffed unit.

We found time to visit the Wasa Museum. This houses the spectacular Royal Warship *Wasa*, which capsized on her maiden voyage in 1628 and was salvaged in 1961. It was a relatively new museum when we went there, but already had attracted large numbers of visitors from many different countries.

Later in the day, I took a boat trip round the harbour of Stockholm, with Mr Heber Langston, a consultant orthopaedic surgeon from Winchester, then Chairman of the BMA Consultants' Committee whose knowledge of Sweden was far greater than mine.

Sweden spends a higher percentage of its national income on welfare than do the other Scandinavian countries and marginally more than the UK. The relatively low birth rate and long life expectancy in Sweden means that the country will ultimately face one of the greatest old-age problems in the world.

If circumstances led to my living in a country other than my own, I believe that Sweden would be my choice.

PORTUGAL – 1965

We decided to rent an apartment in a farmhouse in Colares near Sintra in the south of Portugal and visited Burgos and Valladolid en route. The pride of Burgos is its thirteenth-century cathedral with ornamental towers, a magnificent rose window and the *Escalera Dorada* (golden staircase) designed in 1519 by Diego de Siloê. The Carthusian monastery of Miraflores, founded in 1441, is where 'Joan the Mad' kept the body of her dead husband 'Phillip the Handsome' for three months, hoping that he would come to life. It may be a recommendation for Spanish wine that it is said that Phillip died in 1506 of a fever produced by drinking a glass of cold water. Not far south is Valladolid, which was at one time the capital of Spain. We stopped for a short time in the main square on a very hot day and missed seeing the Palace of the Vivero, St Gregory's College and the cathedral, hoping to reach the south of Portugal that day.

The roads were quiet, picturesque, and driving was effortless. Driving in Spain on main roads seemed much less stressful than is the case in Great Britain and various other European countries.

Colares is a small village only a few miles north of Lisbon, and about a mile from Sintra, where there is the famous Pena Palace. We could look up at its floodlit silhouette at night. Most days we had a picnic on the beach and a meal in the local restaurant in the evening. It specialised in soups (*sopas*) usually containing garlic, olive oil and perhaps a poached egg.

The language is rather different from Spanish, but one does not need to be a great linguist to appreciate that *sopas* are soups.

Some years later, my deputy, Dr Arnold Seeram, went

with his wife on a coach tour to Portugal. He was a charming man, and an excellent doctor, but tended to put off until tomorrow what need not be done today. When I would ask him if he could do something for me, he invariably agreed, but often qualified his agreement by saying, 'later'. Now the French word for milk is *lait*, the Italian *latte* and the Portuguese *leite*.

When his coach party, mainly consisting of older ladies, was taken to a nightclub, an attentive Portuguese waiter asked him if his party would like drinks.

Dr Seeram, true to form, said, 'Later.'

Of course the waiter thought that he said, '*Leite*.' About half an hour afterwards the perspiring waiter returned bearing a tray with a number of glasses of milk.

'Sorry to be so long,' he said, 'but we seldom get asked for milk in this nightclub, and I had to go to a farm some distance away.'

Our stay at Colares was marred by a rather frightening experience. The flat in the farmhouse had never previously been occupied and was well fitted out, with a separate shower room where the water was heated by bottled gas.

After a day on the beach, we came back for a shower and change before dinner. My wife and I, and then our elder daughter, had showers. Rosalind, the younger daughter, was last. We thought that she was taking rather a long time, so I knocked on the door but got no reply. When I went in, I found her lying unconscious on the floor. The pilot light had blown out and she had been gassed. When we carried her out to the couch, she began to have slight convulsions and for a short time looked moribund.

It was a tremendous relief when she recovered consciousness in a few minutes and asked why we were fussing so much.

We had several interesting excursions from Colares. One was to the *Cabo da Roca*, on the *Costa de Prata* (Silver

Coast), the long central stretch of the Portuguese Atlantic Coast south of the River Douro. The *Cabo de Roca* is the most westerly point in Europe.

Later we went to a bullfight at Cascais. In Portugal, unlike Spain, the bull is not killed. Further south is Estoril, once the seaside resort of the crowned heads of Europe. It has spa facilities and a fine beach which is to some extent spoiled by the fact that the railway line separates it from the main sea front promenade, the *Estrada Marginal*.

Lisbon is quite near and lies on the river Tagus about ten miles inland from the Atlantic. It is impossible to miss the Tower of Belem (Bethlehem) or the Jerônimos Monastery, which started as a chapel for seamen built by Henry the Navigator. Before Vasco da Gama sailed for India in 1497, he prayed there for the success of his mission.

One of the world's largest collections of state coaches is the *Museu Nacional dos Coches*, but I consider that the display in the Kremlin is more impressive.

Crossing the Tagus at Lisbon is the *Ponte Suspensa* or *Ponte do 25 de Abril*. It was opened in 1966, so was almost complete at the time of our visit.

On the return journey we travelled north through the university city of Coimbra, then Porto (Oporto), on the river Douro. It has many British connections, with British names on the warehouses, and has a particularly fine monument of Henry the Navigator.

We stayed the night at Pontevedra, just north of the Portuguese-Spanish border, a picturesque granite town with arcaded streets and many old houses bearing armorial shields. About the size of Eastbourne, it is attractively situated on the *Ria de Pontevedra*, the estuary of the rivers Lêrez, Alba and Tomeza.

We went to an open air fête, with music and dancing until it was time for dinner, which often in some parts of Spain is not served till ten at night.

Going further north, we soon reached Santiago de Compostella, celebrated throughout the world as a centre of pilgrimage with a very fine cathedral. The shrine of the Apostle St James, the patron saint of Spain, is where his bones were buried after his martyrdom in AD 44. Having an interest in pharmacology, I visited the Faculty of Pharmacy in the Colegio Fonseca, built in 1544.

There was a good road – now a motorway – to La Coruna on the north coast. It is famous in English history as Corunna. It was here, in the Peninsula War (1809), that Sir John Moore's army fought a gallant rearguard action. Moore was mortally wounded but did not die until he had heard that the embarkation of his troops was successful.

Being on the north-west coast it is exposed to the Atlantic winds and characteristic features are the *mirandores* (glazed balconies) which provide protection.

We continued along the north coast, often on winding roads with heavy lorry traffic until we reached the *Cuevas de Altamira* (Caves of Altamira) containing prehistoric paintings of the upper Magdalenian Age – about 12,000 BC. There are drawings of bisons, boar and deer painted in orchre. I bought an inexpensive print.

Whenever I have travelled abroad I have bought a wooden coathanger – and later inscribed its origin in poker work – and a print, both inexpensive and easy to carry.

I carried a piece of string with a knot about two thirds along its length, so that I could measure a print and ensure that it would fit into my flight bag without being bent. When I bought a Munch print in Oslo, the shopkeeper was obviously puzzled when he saw me looking at the prints and then measuring their length and breadth. As you can imagine, our house is full of wooden coathangers and prints. One print which I particularly like, is a Remington depicting an Indian on horseback. This I bought in the Chicago Art Museum for one dollar. I believe that the former American President, Lyndon Johnson, had a fine collection of Remington's original works.

After the visit to the caves at Altamira, we returned home and hope to go back some day.

FINLAND – JUNE 1966

In 1966 the International Hospital Federation Study Tour was in Finland and I was privileged to join the group. We started at the capital, Helsinki, staying at the Marski Hotel, where I had my first sauna. Helsinki has a population of about 500,000. To gain an impression of the city, one can take a tram ride. It had an excellent 3T tram which describes a rough figure of eight throughout the city, and now has a new underground train system deep in the city's granite foundations.

The main railway station won a prize for architecture when it was first built. Railway stations can be most elegant structures, as in Rome. Just opposite, is the statue of Mannerheim – a venerated figure in Finland.

We had an excellent guide, the deputy Secretary of the Finnish Medical Association, and set off northwards by coach through Porvoo. There we visited the interesting fifteenth-century cathedral with attractive frescoes and a statue of Alexander I, who appointed the first legislative assembly in 1809.

The road soon skirts the Russian border. On their watchtowers the Russian frontier guards with powerful binoculars, would telephone their opposite numbers in Finland and say, 'Confiscate the Minolta camera being used by the Japanese tourist' and this was done forthwith. This procedure is no longer taking place.

Lapeenranta, founded in 1649, with a population of about 55,000 is the southern terminal for Saimaa lake traffic. At one time it was the centre of a very profitable tar trade. Our guide told us about the wood-burning lake steamer, struggling against the current as it negotiated a curved waterway between two lakes.

'Quickly' shouted the skipper to the engineer below, 'throw some curved logs on the fire.'

After visiting the hospital at Lapeenranta, we continued northwards towards Savonlinna – a fair distance, but with good company and a small refrigerator stocked with drinks, the time passed quickly.

However, what goes in has to come out, so our tactful mentor stopped the bus and said, 'We will now picka mushrooms. The ladies will picka mushrooms on the left side of the road and the gentlemen will picka mushrooms on the right side of the road.'

At Savonlinna I became involved in a discussion with an American administrator and was late for the hospital sauna. So I went this time to the municipal sauna, which is gas-fired, unlike the hospital saunas which were usually heated by electricity.

After sweating it out in the heat and throwing ladles of water on to the hot 'coal', I was lightly beaten by an old woman with a kind of witch's broom.

Meals at the hospital were first class and the staff were invariably kind and welcoming.

Then on to Kuopio where we got superb views from the tower on Puijo Hill. Once again, the hospital was most impressive. Here, as elsewhere in Finland, virtually all the patients were Finnish, whereas in other countries one would find various nationalities amongst the patients.

From Kuopio we went on to Jyväskylä, now going southwards. Its university was designed by Alvar Aalto, the world-famous architect. When we had completed the tour of the hospital I went to the hotel and found to my surprise that Bodkin Adams was staying there. He was at a clay pigeon shooting competition.

Then down to Tampere (pop. 170,000), Finland's second city. It is really an industrial centre and I was told that a Scot, James Finlayson, built the first cotton mill there in

1820. Tampere has a 500 foot observation tower in which is a planetarium, aquarium and children's zoo. It is rather like the Post Office Tower in London, the Euromast in Rotterdam, or the needle in Seattle.

As Finland is a relatively flat country in the south, one does not often get many views but the vista from the Näsinneula Tower was superb.

A number of the long stretches of road were not covered by tarmac, so tended to be dusty in summer and muddy in winter. However, a chemical substance was devised which would bind the mud like concrete; unfortunately it had a tendency to cause the underneath of a car to rust.

'So,' our mentor said, 'We Finns have to choose between dust and rust.'

A psychiatric hospital in that area gave us a very favourable impression of the standards of care for the mentally ill. A wooden wool spindle, beautifully carved, remains with me as a souvenir of my visit to the hospital occupational therapy department.

We were now on our way back to Helsinki prior to returning to the UK. As I had never visited Oslo I decided to leave the day before the main party and make my own way there, being able to get the air ticket re-routed.

Oslo has so much of interest that it was impossible to see much in half a day – but again I was able to take photographs of the royal castle, the castle guard, the harbour and so on.

By pure chance, in the lift going up to my room in the evening in the Oslo hotel, I met two Americans who told me that the Scandinavian Air Service were on strike. So I set my alarm, got up at 4.00 a.m. and walked several miles to the airport. The only British plane was fully booked but I persuaded the airport manager to write 'Re-routed due to strike' on my ticket. Then I had the good fortune to meet a Norwegian farmer, dressed in dungarees, who had a small

Cessna plane. With some difficulty, including language problems, I persuaded him to take me to Copenhagen. By law, a plane flying out of the country has to have a co-pilot, and again fortune smiled on me, because I met an SAS pilot on strike who wanted to go there.

Two stranded Russians and an American joined us and we took off. The Norwegian had never previously flown outside Norway but the SAS pilot navigated whilst I sat behind him reading the map and being fumigated by Russian cigarettes.

We were ordered to land right out on the periphery at Taastrup Airport, Copenhagen, and found the main airport lounge crowded with anxious travellers unable to get away.

So I went round all the various desks and got various opinions – Lufthansa said fly to Hamburg and take a train, KLM could take me to Amsterdam but I had no money left for extra travelling expenses. Finally I tried Aer Lingus who had a charter flight about to leave for Manchester. Fortunately for me, one of the party had failed to turn up after his night out in Copenhagen, so I was able to have his seat – and a generous free sample of Irish whiskey en route.

At Manchester airport I got a shuttle to Heathrow, Tube to Victoria and train to Eastbourne, arriving just in time to attend the medical staff committee meeting where I wanted to present some special project I had been working on.

Finland was a delightful country although its language, more akin to Hungarian than Scandinavian, was difficult to understand. If I had stayed with the main party this would have been no problem. I was astounded by the high standard of medical care, bearing in mind that the Finns had had to pay vast sums in reparations to Russia at the end of the war. Yet it seemed to be doing just as well as Sweden which had had no such handicap.

The relative cost of living then was high. The currency is

the mark, about eight to the pound sterling, with 100 penniäa (singular penni) to the mark.

But the visitor can get low-priced accommodation in boarding houses (*matkustajakooti*).

The food in hospitals and hotels was excellent: *poronkieltä* (reindeer tongues with lemon sauce), *poron karistys* (reindeer casserole) and *kalakukko* (fish and pork baked in a rye flour crust, and a speciality of Kuopio), and the memorable Finnish liqueurs – *lakka* (Cloudberry) and *mesimarja* (Arctic bramble), which are quite delicious and unlike any other liqueur.

Now my main idea is to return and see more of this fascinating country.

NORWAY – JUNE 1966

My knowledge of Norway is limited to visiting Oslo and learning about the country from Norwegian friends. Many of the 4,000,000 inhabitants are involved directly or indirectly with fishing. Norway is one of Europe's leading fishing nations. But now the oil finds in the North Sea have affected Norway in a similar way to Aberdeen. Although mineral resources are relatively small, the Norwegians have developed hydro-electric power extremely well. About half the population live in the south-east, including 500,000 in Oslo.

Scenically, Norway is one of the most dramatic countries in the world, its fjords attracting many tourists. Friends of my generation feel less well disposed to a country when they have memories such as Narvik or convoys to Murmansk.

Oslo is probably the most spacious city in the world, with an area of 173,000 square miles – yet the total population is less than 500,000. There are certain affinities in the languages of Denmark, Norway and Sweden.

I could identify the Gamlebyen (the old town) having visited Den Gamle by (the old people's town) in Copenhagen.

Probably the most outstanding building is the City Hall, which rises above Pipervika harbour on Rädhusplass (City Hall Square). It was inaugurated in 1950 for the city's 900th anniversary. There are not many capital cities where one can watch the changing of the guard at the Royal Palace but this takes place every day at 1.40 p.m. in Oslo. Nearby is the cathedral built between 1694 and 1699 and above the harbour is the Renaissance-style Akershus Castle rebuilt on the site of the medieval fortress in the 17th century.

Even on a brief visit it is well worth finding time to see the Viking Ships, the Kon-Tiki raft and the ship used in polar exploration by Nansen and Amundsen – the *Fram*. For the photographer and of course the student of sculpture – there are works by Gustav Vigeland in Frogner Park. I bought a print of a painting by Edvard Munch whose works reflect his childhood dominated by poverty, sickness and death.

My stay in Oslo lasted for less than 24 hours, including four hours' sleep, but I saw enough to leave me with an abiding memory of a beautiful and interesting city.

JUGOSLAVIA

When I was stationed at Lignano Sabbiadoro, south of Trieste in 1945, my friend Arnold Blackwell, who had been O.C. of a Field Dressing Station at Padua, was moved to Pola, now called Pula, in Northern Yugoslavia. Arnold Blackwell was a first-class clinician and administrator. I had no hesitation in recommending him for promotion (Captain to Major) when he was my second-in-command on the Venice Lido. Sadly, he died after a coronary thrombosis while running a busy general practice in Birmingham, after surviving the rigours of the campaign in Italy. He was known as 'Pickles' or 'Senõr Crossan'.

The walls and hoardings were all daubed 'Zivel Tito' – Long Live Tito, and I became increasingly aware of the dominance of this man, Josip Broz, who later took the name of Tito and was President from 1953 until 1980. There is a great deal to be said for adopting a brief, simple name if one wishes to indulge in self advertisement. Hitler sounds better than Schikelgrüber and Stalin better than Dzhugashvili. Age Concern is a better and more easily grasped title than the National Old People's Welfare Council. Parents should always consider the endless explanations which a child will have to give throughout his life if he is christened Christopher Columbus rather than John or Peter. The sister of Florence Nightingale (born in Florence) was called Parthenope – the Greek word for Naples, where she was born. It is also wise to make a few discreet enquiries, lest a child is given an apparently innocuous name which may have a sinister or obscene connotation in another language. The French have unfortunately named a soft drink Pschitt – which illustrates my point.

When I returned to Yugoslavia with my wife and two small girls, we booked in advance a room in a private house through the local tourist information office at Crikvenica, pronounced Tsrikvenitsa, a seaside resort on the Adriatic Coast about 50 miles south of Trieste.

The journey by car involved crossing several frontiers and, in particular, there was a long queue of vehicles at the border between Austria and Yugoslavia. In consequence, we arrived so late that the authorities would not allow us to arouse the tenants of the house where we had booked accommodation. In 1967, especially at midnight, there were not many English-speaking people about, but we finally found a room at the Hotel Therapia, which proved to be an excellent choice.

It is just opposite the island of Krk, a pleasant boat trip and interesting place to visit 35 years ago, but now industrialised and rather crowded with tourists. It was under Venetian jurisdiction from the year 1115 until the late 18th century.

The Plitvice Lakes (Plitvicka Jereza), one of Yugoslavia's greatest tourist attractions, were nearby. There are 16 separate lakes and many beautiful waterfalls. Visitors come from far afield – we had to negotiate with a carload of Russians on a one-way piece of road leading to the lakes at the time when repairs to the surface made the one-way traffic system necessary. The traffic control, unfortunately, was not particularly well organised.

We passed country dwellers cooking piglets on spits in the open over wooden fires and found endless subjects for photography. At the lakes, with waters shimmering blue and green there are brilliantly coloured dragonflies hovering over the waterfalls.

In Crickvenica there are relics of a Roman settlement Ad Tures and an interesting church. The word *crickva* is Yugoslav for church. We spent quite a time admiring an old lady crocheting lace in the main square and I bought a bottle of the local fire-water called *sljivovica* – plum brandy.

Back at the hotel, where the bedroom floor was varnished wood, the bottle got knocked over and the contents completely removed the varnish. So we took it well diluted.

During our stay the weather was good, with a dry warm wind called the *bura*. In the winter the cold wind is called *yugu*, and there is a *maestral* like the French *mistral*.

The Yugoslavs eat a snack called *burek*, a greasy Turkish-style pastry which can be obtained from a street kiosk with cheese (*sa sirom*), meat (*sa mesom*) or apple (*sa jabukama*). The children liked the ice-cream parlours (*slasticuarnica*).

We did not manage to visit the capital – Belgrade (Beograd) 'The White City' nor Ljubljana where Tito was based during the war. In spite of wartime memories, there were many German nationals on holiday in the area. Yet whole villages had been wiped out by the Nazis. One of the many lessons I learned during my travels is that we must always look forward and not harbour grudges.

Optimism must be the keynote – I firmly believe that the world is becoming a better place and that within a generation we shall no longer think of Russia as a potential enemy.

NORTH AMERICA – AUGUST 1967

My first visit to North America was with the International Hospital Federation in August, 1967. It was an exciting prospect and I was full of enthusiasm when I was about to go aboard an Air Canada plane at Heathrow.

'I'm afraid there is no seat for you,' the stewardess said, 'Our computers shows that every seat in the aircraft is occupied.'

Fortunately, after I had flourished my air ticket, the stewardess made a phone call and was told that there had been a computer error or more likely a human error and the seat was available.

As the plane approaches Canada, one can get a fine view of the southern tip of Greenland and of the icebergs, so I lost no time in taking a few photographs.

On this occasion, I was paired with the House Governor of Moorfields Eye Hospital, a Mr Green, who was a most interesting and delightful companion. On arrival at Montreal, we went to our hotel where I asked the black desk clerk for our room key.

'My colleague here is Green,' said I, 'and I'm Brown.'

Without batting an eyelid, the clerk handed over the key saying, 'You guys have sure got your own colour problem to resolve.'

We visited the Montreal General Hospital, noticing *en route* the prevailing French names of streets and districts – Maisonneuve, Outremont, Côte St Luc. The road around Montreal International Airport is Boulevard Mêtropolitain.

The hospital provided a high standard of care. One of the ways of assessing this is to study patients' case notes. I was concerned to learn that victims of street accidents are ultimately billed for the cost of ambulance transport to the hospital – the ambulance service there being a private concern rather like a taxi service. Perhaps we have gone to the other extreme in Britain, where an ambulance may call to collect a patient for day hospital treatment – free of transport charges – to be told that the patient is out shopping.

We then went to Toronto, where I visited the children's hospital, said to be the best in North America. I had written a paper on the health of hospital staff and looked up all the available references in world literature. One was an article written by Hunnisett, Children's Hospital, Toronto.

Mr Hunnisett received me with great courtesy, and I gave him a reprint of my *Lancet* article of 19th December, 1964.

'Your name is fairly common in East Sussex, England, where I work,' I explained.

'Not surprising,' was the reply, 'My parents emigrated to Canada from Westham, near Pevensey, and I was born here.'

He had considerable ability and was the Chief Administrator of the hospital.

Our group then visited a hospital at the time under construction at Scarborough, quite near Toronto. It was being built to a very high standard and was very different from the old workhouse, St Mary's Hospital in Eastbourne.

That night we stayed in a hotel at Niagara Falls. In the town was a sign which said, 'Ears pierced while you wait'. In the evening before dinner we had a swim in the hospital pool, which seemed to me to be surprisingly warm. This I took to be the pattern in North America. When I enquired of the hotel manager, he seemed surprised and was not too pleased to learn that a small boy had turned up the thermostat to its maximum.

Millions of tourists visit the falls, those on the Canadian side of the border being the bigger, to the discomfiture of some Americans. Crossing the border between Canada and America was an incredible experience. The amount of form filling was enormous – it was necessary to record one's mother's date of birth and so on. I was astounded by the amount of resources being allocated to the elaborate formalities required to cross over from Canada to America – it all seemed a pointless waste of time and indeed there are endless opportunities of crossing the border other than at the recognised checkpoints without any form of documentation. It was a worse experience than crossing at Checkpoint Charlie in Berlin.

Our next stop was Detroit, where we had opportunities of visiting the facilities at Ann Arbor University and the vast Henry Ford museum, with its infinitely varied collection of automobiles and railway engines, bigger than any I had ever seen before.

I had many problems with the American language. Because drinks at the bar were relatively expensive, we of the British contingent became accustomed to foregathering in one or other of our bedrooms for a drink before dinner. Now it so happened that I had bought a bottle of American whiskey – there are numerous brands such as Old Kentucky, etc. – but I happened to have bought a bottle of Old Crow.

So just before dinner, Sir Albert Martin, chairman of a hospital board, invited me to have a drink with him.

'That is most kind of you, sir, but as a matter of fact I have some Old Crow up in my bedroom.'

He looked at me rather strangely and never spoke to me again.

From Detroit we flew to Rochester, Minnesota, to visit the Mayo Clinic. On arrival at Rochester Airport we were told that there might be some delay because of difficulty in getting our baggage unloaded.

After we had sat in a coach for about an hour – it was

about 10.00 p.m. – I approached the black coach driver and said, 'Surely you must be loaded by this time of night.'

'No, man,' he replied, 'Ah'm a teetotaller.'

At the Mayo Clinic I was able to make what I was told was a unique comment. Each consultant had coloured buttons on his desk which would illuminate coloured light bulbs in the corridor outside his door. Blue for a laboratory technician, green for a nurse, red for a secretary, yellow for a radiographer and so on. When I asked what would happen if one of them happened to be colour-blind, I was told that no one had ever previously asked this question.

More language problems beset me in Chicago. The city was then the only place in the world with two Hilton Hotels, the original Conrad Hilton and Palmer House in State Street.

When I booked in at Palmer House, I was given the key to room 1728, that is, room 28 on the 17th floor. When I opened the door, I found to my surprise a quantity of ladies' underclothes on the bed, a suitcase marked Oslo and quite an amount of valuable jewellery on the dressing table. So I phoned reception. No apology was offered, but I was told that I should have been given the key to 1828 on the floor above. So down I went in the elevator, not the lift, and collected the key to 1828.

It proved to be a very fine room with a magnificent view over Chicago, comfortable furnishings, television, etc. but no bed. Again I phoned reception.

'We're very crowded with the conference. You are in part of a suite and the bedroom has been let off separately. But I'll send you a bed.'

Very soon a big black porter appeared with a divan bed, pushed aside the furniture and all seemed well. Then I opened my flight bag which contained one suit and one shirt, but there was nowhere to hang them. Once more a call to reception, explaining that I could not hammer a nail in the wall of such a beautiful room even if I had a nail or hammer.

'You wanna closet?'

'No, I've already been.'

'Aw, you guys in England talk about a wardrobe.'

Again the porter returned, with a chrome-plated clothes rack with 24 metal hangers, standing on four small wheels. So I hung my one suit on a hanger and got into bed. But before I had gone to sleep the porter returned with a metal hat stand – I had no hat.

On the following evening we had a reception in the Palmer House Hotel where I was introduced to the daughter of the President of the American Medical Association, who came from the deep south. So I told her my true story of what had happened the previous night prompting her to explain that she had a lady friend living in Switzerland who wanted to visit the deep south. Now the people in that area are very religious and have Wayside Chapels where they can stop to say a prayer – sometimes there are 200 or 300 miles between townships. On the maps the presence of a Wayside Chapel is shown by the capital letters 'WC.'

When the Swiss girl wrote to book a room in a hotel, she asked that it should have a room with a nice view, a comfortable bed, a separate shower and by the way she wrote, 'Is there a WC?'

The manager replied, 'Madame, we look forward to welcoming you to our hotel of which we are very proud. You can have a room with a fine view, a really comfortable bed and a shower. With reference to the WC there is an excellent one, admittedly seven miles down the road, but there is a very good bus service.'

GERMANY DUSSELDORF – JUNE 1969

The second occasion on which I represented the British Medical Association at a meeting of the International Hospital Federation was in 1959. The IHF customarily held a congress and a study tour on alternate years and 1959 was the year of a congress which was held at Dusseldorf.

It is the banking and administrative centre of the Rühr with a population of about 750,000. Although badly damaged by bombing, it has been rebuilt and is now a prosperous industrial centre on the Rhine. A small part of the original old town remains and there one can get small boys to do cartwheels (*radschlagen*) by throwing a mark on the pavement. This is a prized relic of past customs, like the blowing of the horn by the watchman in Ripon.

The Germans are an industrious hard-working people on the whole, apart from some of the youth, who like some youth in other countries such as Britain are parasites and a sad reflection on their forebears who sacrificed so much. A feeling of bitterness pervades after visiting a military cemetery, where lie one's friends killed when only in their early twenties.

Millions of Jews were massacred for no other reason than that they were Jewish.

We spent some time in the oldest part of Dusseldorf where there are many seventeenth- and eighteenth- century houses surviving and the crooked spire of the church of St Lambertus is a notable landmark.

It is in this area where the young lads turn cartwheels. The tradition goes back to the wedding of Elector Johan Wilhelm in the seventeenth century. When a wheel of the wedding coach became loose, a ten-year-old boy saved the situation by attaching himself to the wheel and cartwheeling with it to the end of the parade.

Our meetings were held in the Messehalle not far from the hotel and we enjoyed our early morning walk to get there along the river bank. From my hotel room before 8.00 in the morning, I could see water carts washing the streets and workers busy in adjacent offices. Even after the war, the Germans seem sensitive to authority. We noticed that at a time when there was no traffic in sight, pedestrians would not cross the road when the lights were red.

I had memories of being struck on the arm by a policeman's baton in Chicago because I put one foot off the sidewalk whilst hurrying to a meeting.

In Belgium, as one might expect, crossing the road even empty of traffic with lights at red brought a mild reprimand from the gendarme, '*Soyez prudent, monsieur.*'

After the conference and exhibition, I went to West Berlin and stayed in the Schweitzerhof Hotel, which was very conveniently situated. Having read so much about Berlin, I was fascinated to see it in reality. About 2,000,000 people lived in West Berlin, and one million in East Berlin, separated of course, by the notorious wall. There was no real problem for the tourist crossing over, although one tended to be shown the better aspects of East Berlin. But after all, wherever one goes, the official party is shown what is most favourable and, although it is interesting, I have found that going it alone can sometimes be rather difficult and even dangerous.

In West Berlin, we visited the Stieglitz Clinic, a modern showpiece with high technology medicine. In the hospital canteen there were no staff. By selecting a menu, and putting a coin in a machine, the meal appears on disposable plates with disposable cutlery, which is left in the rubbish bin. This was something I had never seen before, and it was most impressive.

It was my responsibility to visit the British Military Hospital at Charlottenberg, a suburb of Berlin, to find out how the young army doctors were faring. The hospital was built by the Germans and has an underground replica of the above ground hospital, to provide self-contained accommodation in the event of a nuclear war. Naturally, the service personnel stationed in Berlin were fit men, so the workload was light. We were able to discuss the possibility of our army doctors working part time in German civil hospitals, but this presented various problems.

At night one can always use as a guiding beacon the rotating Mercedes sign on a high building, although after a long day walking round hospital wards, one was glad to get to bed early.

I would have liked to have spent more time in Germany, but learnt a great deal in the relatively short itinerary.

DUBLIN – JUNE 1971

Vikings founded Dublin and there are still buildings surviving from their ninth- and tenth- century occupation. The name Dublin means Black Pool, from the peat-stained waters of the River Liffey. For a few moments I thought that my life was in danger, when to open a conversation, I asked one of the university professors if he was a native of Blackpool. But of course he was a professor in the faculty of medicine, who had not had the benefits of a wide education like his colleagues in the department of arts.

It is somewhat presumptuous of me to write about Dublin, because I have been there on only two occasions, once for a BMA meeting in 1952 and once in June 1971 for a meeting of the International Hospital Federation.

When I took the train from Euston, I occupied one of two seats at a table in the restaurant car, and was joined by the late Emmanuel Shinwell. He was easily recognisable as he had been photographed on so many occasions in his long parliamentary career. Like all politicians I have met, he was a great talker and I thought that he must have been vaccinated with a gramophone needle. Admittedly, I was somewhat overawed but I did not manage to interject more than a few sentences before we reached Holyhead. Undoubtedly, he was a brilliant debater or, rather, orator. Britain had gained immeasurably from Jewish immigrants – as an avid reader of biographies of such eminent men as the Grades, Guttman of Stoke Mandeville and numerous others I have come to appreciate their immense contribution to our society. It may be that a significant reason for the paramount position of the United States of America is that it has so many talented immigrants. At no time during my visit to Russia did I meet an immigrant who had made a major contribution to the Russian state.

As in the USA, I was faced with language difficulties. My room was in an excellent boarding house in Dun Laoghaire – but no one could tell me where to find Dun Layhoch Hair. Fortunately, I encountered a fluent linguist who advised me to look for Dun Leery.

My first hospital visit was to both the old and new St Vincent's – the latter a real showpiece although, as usual, there were regrets from the Senior Staff about leaving the old building.

The Irish have a great sense of tradition. Indeed I was told that the General Post Office in Dublin is regarded as a kind of shrine of Irish patriotism. O'Connell Street somehow reminded me of Princes Street in Edinburgh, although I admit they are not at all similar. I spent quite a time in Trinity College and brought back photographs of the Bank of Ireland opposite – that's where the real power lies, I was told. My informant did not explain what he meant by the word 'lies'. I had heard so much of the famous Rotunda Maternity Hospital that I had to see it and was shown round by a phlebotomist – we call such a person a blood transfusion doctor in our simple way. He was an Irish graduate and an excellent guide, raconteur and presumably a good phlebotomist. Apart from telling me about his job he told me about the man who went into a bar in Northern Ireland leading a crocodile by a piece of string.

'Do you serve Catholics here?' he asked the barman. The barman said he did. 'Good, then I'll have a pint of beer for meself and a Catholic for the crocodile.'

Rather than starting a discussion about religion, I talked about crocodiles.

Two explorers were crossing the depths of Central Africa and quenched their thirst on the local brew.

They decided to cool off by sitting on the jetty by the side of a crocodile-infested river, when suddenly one of them shouted, 'A crocodile has bitten off one of my legs!'

141

'Which one?' said his friend.

'I don't know,' replied the victim, 'all crocodiles look alike to me.'

On the subject of losing a leg you may know that the Earl of Uxbridge at the battle of Waterloo, in 1815, lost his right leg while riding off the field beside the Duke of Wellington.

He said to Wellington, 'By God sir, I've lost my leg.'

The Duke replied 'So you have.'

When a descendant, a century later, boasted that his ancestor had lost his leg at Waterloo, he received the reply 'Which platform?'

The hospital doctor, with his mind on midwifery, told me that at a recent public lecture on the vast growth in the world population, the lecturer said, 'Each minute, somewhere in this world, a woman gives birth to a child. What can we do?'

Voice from the back of the hall, 'Find that woman and stop her.'

My reaction was to talk about another 'Voice from the back of the hall.' A temperance lecturer had a glass of water and a glass of gin. When he dropped a live worm into the water, it wriggled about. When he dropped it into the gin, it died instantly.

'Now,' he said to his audience, 'what does this prove?'

Voice from the back – 'If you've got worms, drink gin.'

It was not my choice to revert to religious topics, but the phlebotomist told me about the Irish priest who was visiting the Pope.

When His Holiness said, 'Have I seen you before?' the priest said 'No,' whereupon the Pope said, 'Then you must have a double.'

'Thank you, blessed Father,' said the priest.

The Rotunda impressed me enormously and just as Oxford and Cambridge attract the best brains in the academic world, so the Rotunda is, if I may be permitted to indulge in religious confusion, the Mecca for would-be obstetricians.

Out and about in Dublin, I strolled past the public buildings and town houses built by wealthy aristocrats in the elegant Georgian period before the American revolution. Dublin was battered by the invasions of Cromwell and William of Orange, when it was taken over in the eighteenth century by a new ruling class of Protestant landowners, known as the Anglo-Irish ascendancy, who moved into the city to run the Irish Parliament in its fine building on College Green. Amongst the many fine buildings they created was Leinster House, a prototype for the United States White House.

The official Gaelic title for the Prime Minister, Taoiseach, is pronounced 'tea shook'. When I was told this I was reminded of the man who was a guest in a monastery for one night, and the customary Latin greeting between monks was *Dominus Tecum* – God be with you.

In the morning, one of the monks knocked on his door at reveille and said, '*Dominus Tecum.*'

'Thank you,' said the guest – a Greek rather than Latin scholar? – 'Put it down outside the door and I'll fetch it in a few moments.'

The kindliness and hospitality extended to the Englishman is quite remarkable. Just as the Jamaicans seem to have forgiven the English for their behaviour in the past, so the Irish never reminded me that it was only in 1921 that six Republican prisoners were executed by the English. And there was far less justification for such action then than there is today – these men never committed terrible atrocities such as we have witnessed during the past 30 years.

Meeting in Trinity College was in surroundings so interesting that it was tempting to spend more time studying the college than listening to the speakers. The oldest existing buildings date from the turn of the seventeenth century – a southern Irish colleague reproving me for playing truant from the lectures told me that Trinity Fellows made up in bad manners for what they lacked in training – so I tried to maintain my best behaviour even if I were outside instead of being inside.

The 300-foot Palladian facade dates from 1752–9 when the city of Dublin, with a population of 150,000 was the largest in the British Isles apart from London. The dining hall has portraits of Trinity men – who include Goldsmith, Congreve, Swift, Wilde and Edward Carson. The Trinity library was begun in 1712 and opened in 1732. It contains nearly 1,000,000 manuscripts and is entitled by Act of Parliament to a free copy of every book published in Britain and Ireland. Most visitors make for the Book of Kells compiled in the middle of the eighth century, perhaps the best known of the early Celtic manuscripts.

Oscar Wilde's father was a surgeon who lived in Merrion Square, Dublin's Harley Street – in the vicinity of Fitzwilliam Square.

It is perhaps a sad reflection on my character that I chose to visit the Guinness Brewery instead of exploring further the architectural gems of the city centre. And it may be that more expatriates are familiar with its products than they are with the Book of Kells. It is always fascinating to see a world-famous institution even if it is a brewery. Covering sixty acres, it takes a fair time to traverse and few of the real boozers reckon it is worth the long walk primarily to get a small measure of the real stuff before leaving.

The Irish people are most likeable and it is a great tragedy that the troubles in Ulster make the news, when there is so much goodness abounding in Eire, about which little is heard.

The new Abbey Theatre has a worldwide reputation – the name of Bernard Shaw is well known in such diverse places as Moscow and Bangkok.

Whether you are interested in Renoir, Manet, Degas or in Picasso, Utrillo or Jack Yeats, you will find them all represented in Charlemont House, the Municipal Gallery of Modern Arts.

The hospitals vary from the ultra-modern St Vincent's to the Kilmainham Royal Hospital, which was built in 1680, before the Royal Hospital at Chelsea. It is now a folk museum. The few psychiatrists in our party went to St Patrick's Hospital, known now as Swift's Hospital. He endowed it in his will and wrote:

> He gave the little wealth he had
> To build a house for fools and mad;
> To show by one satiric touch,
> No nation wanted it so much.

For no obvious reason, when I read this I cast my mind back to my arrival in Eastbourne when the proceedings of the town council were printed in our local paper. St Mary's Hospital was then administered by the local authority and a report of a speech by the mayor said, 'Anyone who is familiar with the work of St Mary's Hospital will realise that a bigger mortuary is essential.'

St Brendan's Hospital is a leading centre for geriatric medicine and the James Connolly Hospital has developed its facilities for the elderly to a remarkable extent in recent years. A senior nursing officer there kindly took me to Dublin Castle, where we were received with the customary Irish hospitality.

If my knowledge of Dublin is superficial it is only because time was too short to see more than a small fraction of its treasures, but I learnt a great deal during my brief visits.

RUSSIA – 1972

Because I had had some experience of international medical meetings, when it was announced that the 9th International Congress of Gerontology was to be held in Kiev in 1972, my colleagues proposed that I should undertake to arrange group travel for the British participants. Fortunately I had got to know Dr Gwendolyn Ayers, Ph.D., retired from a distinguished career in the British Foreign Office. She had asked my advice about material for a book, *England's First State Hospitals 1867–1930*, published by the Wellcome Institute for the History of Medicine and although I had in fact helped her to a very minor extent, she agreed to help me arrange the visit to Kiev.

This involved almost daily telephoning and letter writing for more than a year, dealing with Aeroflot and Intourist, so that ultimately we chartered a Russian TU 104 to go from Gatwick Airport with 101 passengers. For the majority of the group, it was their first visit to the Soviet Union and the Russians had done everything possible to make us feel welcome. We were aware of some of the differences between the Ukraine and other parts of the USSR. Although the percentage of elderly persons in the Soviet Union is considerably less than in many other countries, including Great Britain, the Ukrainians have taken a special interest in the ageing process and are justifiably proud of their Institute of Gerontology.

Apart from the time spent in preparatory organisation, virtually all of which was done by Dr Ayers, I tried to make myself familiar with Russian each morning as I was shaving, by studying the Cyrillic alphabet, which I had written on a placard on the bathroom wall. I had learned to use time in this way from my school headmaster who used to say that he learned Spanish whilst shaving. This in no way implies that only beardless men can learn languages.

Also I joined the Society for Cultural Relations with the USSR. The chairman was Dr Leonard Crome, MC, FRCP, who had been with me in the field ambulance in North Africa. He won the MC at Cassino and was fluent in several languages. Born in Russia, he had taken part in the Spanish Civil War, having graduated in medicine in Edinburgh in 1934. I had spent a week's leave with him in Rome in 1944 and he gave me invaluable advice about the USSR before we went to the conference in 1972.

The Journal of the Society published my impressions of the meeting in its edition of December 1972, when I was able to describe the opening of the Congress in the Ukrainia Palace which easily accommodated the 3,000 or so delegates, plus their wives and children who probably accounted for a further 1,500. The speeches of welcome by the president Professor D. F. Chebotarev, of the USSR, and Professor Nathan Shock of the USA were listened to with great respect.

We had to overcome certain difficulties before leaving the UK. It so happened that in the early part of 1972, a number of Russian diplomats were expelled from this country, which did nothing to ease our negotiations with Intourist and Aeroflot, both of which are official state agencies. Also, *The Times* published an advertisement under the heading 'Famous Last Words' – 'Your Next Conference Could Be Your Last' designed to emphasise the importance of choosing the best conference organiser and we were, of course, complete amateurs.

Meanwhile I persevered with Russian language tapes, although I found it difficult in the short time I had to spare from routine hospital work to make much headway. Visitors to the USSR should try to familiarise themselves with the Russian alphabet and learn a few simple phrases such as *dobraye utra* (good day), *dubri vyecher* (good evening), *spasibo* (thank you), *da* (yes), *niet* (no), *nichivo* (it doesn't matter).

Our departure from Gatwick went quite smoothly, although we noticed the somewhat Victorian décor of the interior of the TU 104. The pressurisation mechanism differed from other planes I had known, in particular when clouds of vapour appeared in the cabin. I tried to keep my companions interested by telling them about the two professors of medicine who were crossing the Atlantic in a plane with two seats on the left side of the aisle and three seats on the right. When a lady with two young children went forward to the toilets amidships, she pushed the little boy into the left toilet and went herself into the right-hand toilet accompanied by the little girl.

It was obvious that the boy had no need to use the toilet, as he came out after a few seconds and returned to his seat.

Seeing the toilet vacant one of the professors went forward and entered.

Soon after, the lady came out of the right-hand toilet, tapped on the opposite door and said, 'Don't forget your zipper,' then resumed her seat.

When the professor rejoined his colleague, he said 'The service on these airlines is really first class. These air stewardesses think of everything.'

Then I told them about the modest lady who covered the windows of the aircraft toilet with newspaper, so that no one could look in from outside whilst she was in a state of undress.

She had nervously said to the stewardess before boarding the plane, 'Do these planes crash often?' to which question the stewardess replied, 'No madam, only once.'

The reference to newspapers recalled my experience when travelling by train in this country. My fellow passenger sitting opposite me in the compartment was reading a newspaper and, as he completed each page, he threw it out of the window. After half an hour of this bizarre routine, I asked politely why the pages of newspaper were being cast out of the carriage window.

'To keep away the elephants,' he said.

'But there are no elephants.'

'Of course not,' he replied, 'This demonstrates how well my scheme works.'

Small talk like this may seem to some to be irritating. Somerset Maugham, writing of the Bröntes said, 'Emily was too shy to take part in it and was irritated by those who did. She had no patience with social small talk, which of course is for the most part, trivial; it is merely an expression of general amiability and people take part in it because they have good manners.'

We arrived in Kiev as planned, and the next morning the Congress opened at the October Palace of Culture with a series of papers on Modern Ideas on the Essence of Ageing.

My paper was entitled 'Social and Medical Problems caused by large-scale movement of elderly folk to UK south coast resorts.' The term we had coined – the *Costa Geriatrica* – to describe the area was appreciated by the Spanish and French delegates, but the Japanese and Russians sat impassively.

It so happened that one Sunday morning in Eastbourne I had been at the garage for petrol when I met the late Cyril Connolly. We engaged in small talk but when I mentioned the term *Costa Geriatrica*, he reproved me for mixing the Latin and Greek roots, pointing out that the term should be *Costa Senilis*.

During the discussion following my paper, it emerged that an entirely different problem was facing those concerned with the elderly in Israel. There, the vast majority (96%) of their old people were immigrants, coming from 80 countries, among them the United

Kingdom and the USSR. One of the greatest difficulties was in communication because 60% of those aged 74 and over did not leave their country of origin until they were over 60 years of age. Naturally, many were unable to learn the language of their new home – Hebrew.

Some of the Russian speakers claimed that there was considerable longevity in parts of their country. It was said that one man was 167 years old, which means that he was a child at the time of Napoleon's retreat from Moscow. Various reasons were suggested to account for this longevity – the rural as opposed to urban life, diet, rare herbs and so on, but no one denied that there was an absence of birth records 100 years ago. All the papers were printed in abstract form and issued later to the delegates in three volumes.

We are accustomed to read criticism of Russia in our press. When I was invited to visit the Russian cultural attaché in Kiev, he produced a copy of *Pravda*, with a front page centre photograph of British troops in Northern Ireland aiming rifles at civilians and by implication, shooting their own countrymen.

'We do not behave like this in Russia,' said the cultural attaché.

Could I have done anything else but remain silent?

The inaugural meeting was held in a vast hall with representatives from many other countries of the world and various receptions were arranged, to enable views to be exchanged as far as language barriers would permit.

It had been decided to return to Britain via Moscow, where we were to spend a couple of days sightseeing. On the last day of the conference, we went to the ballet in Kiev, to see Prokofiev's *Romeo and Juliet*. It was an unforgettable experience, demonstrating without a doubt the superiority of the Russians in this form of art. I carried with me a relatively sophisticated IBM tape recorder which

I held on my knees throughout the performance, recording the highlights.

We were due to leave Kiev the following evening at 6.00 p.m. and duly went to the airport. To my concern the young Intourist Aeroflot guide told me that there would be a four-hour delay in taking off as it was raining in Moscow.

'Surely,' I suggested naively, 'you are accustomed to flying in deep snow in this country and some rain in July should not interrupt your schedules.'

No discussion took place, so I asked if I could use the airport tannoy to inform my colleagues.

'*Niet.*' No.

So I crept behind the reception desk and found a loud hailer, using it to explain that there would be a four-hour delay because of rain in Moscow. The suggestion was so absurd that everyone laughed loudly, although one irate member of our group made a point of telling the guide that the explanation was obviously a cover-up for Soviet incompetence and inefficiency. At this she became very upset, trembled, and seemed near to tears. She told me that her husband, also an Intourist guide, was at the time with a group in Spain, that her baby was with her mother in Kiev and that she was frightened of flying. After four hours we boarded the plane and I sat next to our guide who was still tense and trembling, so I took my tape recorder from my pocket switched it on and held it on my shoulder, a few inches from her ear.

'Surely,' said the guide, 'this is a recording of our Kiev ballet Prokoviev's *Romeo and Juliet.*'

'Yes, I made the recording last night.'

'Oh, that is regarded as a serious offence.'

The recording continued for about 15 minutes, then she expressed her gratitude and said her only remaining worry was the take-off. When I explained that we had taken off ten minutes earlier and were about 10,000 feet up, she seemed amazed.

Of course when we arrived at Moscow airport it was warm and dry, indeed it had not rained for some weeks. We were told that our hotel bookings had been changed, so I had to board the three buses and explain the changes on the intercom. But in the end it was an inspiring sight to see the red star over the Kremlin as we approached Moscow at dawn.

Like Kiev, Moscow is very clean, the streets being washed every morning. The Moscow River is not polluted and there were fishermen on the banks at most times. From our bedroom windows in the vast Moscow Hotel we could see the Moscovites setting off for work in the early morning, on foot, by train and on the underground. Public transport is very inexpensive and there were relatively few automobiles to be seen in 1972.

Going out with my camera to Red Square before breakfast I was greeted affably by many Russian visitors to Moscow on a pilgrimage to Lenin's tomb and was asked all sorts of questions which my very limited knowledge of the Russian language made it difficult to answer. Already I had appreciated the diversity of dialects from the different parts of this vast country. No one questioned me when I carried my tape recorder quite openly inside the Kremlin, with its breathtaking collection of gold stage coaches, furs, jewellery and furniture which had belonged to the Tsars.

We were due to leave Moscow early on the Saturday evening and it was, to say the least, disconcerting when our guide told me that our departure had been postponed until the following day. Once again she gave no reason and indeed almost certainly did not know why there should be further delay.

My colleagues were in the restaurant having their evening meal and there was no tannoy available. So I wrote on a placard, 'Intourist Aeroflot now say that we cannot leave until tomorrow,' and carried this round the tables with appropriate immediate comments from the diners. After the meal, I stood on the reception counter and confirmed what I had written on the placard. Action was demanded. We decided to phone the British Embassy from the telephone in Sir Ronald Tonbridge's bedroom, supported by Sir Ferguson Anderson, the big guns of our party, and got through to the Duty Officer in the Russian Embassy. He sounded efficient and helpful, warned us that anything said would be taped by the Russians and asked to explain our call for help. He was brief and knew precisely how such situations should be handled. At 8.00 p.m. on Saturday evening it was quite certain that no Russian official at any level would alter the timing. We must accept the postponement. Next morning our buses set off for Moscow airport, where I was told that we must pay airport tax of one rouble per person. With untarnished naivety I asked why this item had not been listed with many other aspects of the trip, set out in writing during the past year. Of course, no explanation was forthcoming, so Tom Hurst, Secretary of the Edinburgh Royal Infirmary and recently President of the Institute of Hospital Administrators, volunteered to help me to collect one rouble from each member of the party. Fortunately most had some loose kopeks. 100 kopeks equals one rouble, so we were able to hand over to the authorities 101 roubles, leaving us with some change. By now the remainder of the party had gone through the barrier, so Tom and I felt we needed a drink. The only suitable fluid was Russian champagne, stored in refrigerated recesses in the wall behind the bar and quite inexpensive by Western standards, about one pound a bottle. Midday in July in Moscow Airport lounge was not particularly cool, so when I took off the cork, it shot up to the ceiling with a sound like a rifle shot and this is what a large group of

African medical students studying at Moscow University, and awaiting a flight home, thought it to be. So they dived under the tables, whilst our champagne frothed up out of the bottle, leaving about one glassful between Tom and me. We set off to join the others, but at the reception desk I was told that one of us could not return with the party, as the TU 104 carried only 100 passengers. It was, of course totally unproductive to explain that as 101 of us had come to Russia, in the plane, there must be room for 101 to return. By this time I was becoming somewhat impatient and, picking up my two satchels, one full of documents and the other my overnight kit, strode through the gate, to be physically arrested by KGB officials who carried me back to the reception desk. Fortunately I had taken a photostat copy of our group ticket and demanded to show it to the head of Intourist Aeroflot in Moscow. Within seconds, an intelligent personable man speaking perfect English appeared.

'One of you,' he said, 'will have to return via Paris.'

Tom did not hesitate to give up his place and I joined the others steaming in the stationary TU 104 on the runway.

Very soon we took off and within moments the stewardess announced, 'We are not returning to England, we must go to East Berlin to refuel.'

Again no explanation as to how we had made the outward trip without refuelling. At East Berlin where we had to wait for several hours there was obviously latent aggression among some of our party but nothing untoward happened.

At last we were crossing the Channel and I thought that nothing else could possibly go wrong.

Just then the stewardess announced, 'Fasten your seat belts and prepare to land at Heathrow.'

Heathrow? I snatched off my seatbelt, ran down the centre aisle and pushed aside the curtain leading into the flight deck.

'We're *not* going to Heathrow,' I said. 'This is a chartered flight from Gatwick already nearly a day late.'

So the stewardess rapidly advised the pilot in Russian technical terms. He immediately carried out some aerial acrobatics and we landed at Gatwick. Any member of our group will confirm that all I have said really did happen.

Now I want to quote from an article in *The Sunday Times* dated 7th September, 1986 headed 'Two faces of Russia: Honesty on the line of Tragedy, but still the old chicanery and spying'. Disaster strikes top workers on trip of a lifetime – by Louis Branson from Moscow.

The article reads,

> The orchestra played as the *Admiral Nachimov* went down last week, but few of the victims heard it. Most of the four hundred people who lost their lives were jammed into narrow corridors unable to reach the upper decks in the few minutes before the passenger liner sank, after being rammed by a cargo ship whose crew may have been drowned. Unlike the *Titanic* there were no wealthy or famous names amongst the 1,234 people, 346 of them crew, on board the battered 61-year-old liner as it sank in the worst catastrophe in the Soviet Union's maritime history. For many passengers the Black Sea cruise from Odessa to Batuma near the Turkish border was a reward for outstanding work at the factories and offices. Their Trade Unions had paid more than 60% of their fares which ranged from £150 to £300. In the hours before the disaster the holiday-makers had been sightseeing in Novorossiysa, the sun had been beating down fiercely on them all day as they trailed around the town. They visited the fortress built in 1838 and saw the Eternal Flame in memory of the dead of the Second World War. They also heard Fauré's *Requiem* which was composed for war heroes.

It was hardly surprising that by the time the ship set sail in the evening on a calm sea and at a steady 10 knots, the passengers were tired and hundreds took the final decision to go to bed to their cabins or had chosen to stay on the central decks to listen to the ship's orchestra. Although they did not know it, staying awake saved their lives. Just 45 minutes after setting sail, the liner was rocked by a collision. A cargo ship loaded with 41,000 tonnes of grain, ploughed into the liner's forward starboard side, ripping it apart.

In contrast to the *Titanic*'s leisurely descent, the *Admiral Nakimov* sank in less than 8 minutes. There were plenty of lifeboats, but there was no time to catch them. Of the 1,234 people on board the liner, 836 were saved, 29 of them were admitted to hospital, most of them suffering from pneumonia. 11 bodies were recovered, and 292 people remained unaccounted for. The tragedy had only one possible explanation, human error. As a result of the parliamentary investigation handled by a *politburo* member, both captains of the liner and of the cargo ship were arrested and accused of failing to obey safety regulations. There was confusion over which ship was at fault. Under Russian law any cargo ship must give way to a passenger vessel. However, international law says ships are advised to give way to any vessel approaching, as the cargo ship was, heading towards them on a direct collision course. 'We had radioed a warning,' he said. 'After a pause the radio operator on the other vessel replied, "Don't worry", yet after several minutes we had to repeat our call. Moments later the ships collided.' The possibility that the crew members of one or both of the ships had been drinking is not far-fetched. Despite the crackdown on alcoholism by Michel Gorbachev, the Soviet leader, sailors still go on drinking sprees when they put into port. A newspaper in the Soviet Union recently claimed that many captains and navigators were frequently drunk during voyages. The death toll would have been far higher if the ships had collided further from the shore. The first rescue team were able to cover the seven miles to the collision within eleven minutes. In less than an hour 64 rescue boats were plucking survivors from the warm sea. Ten helicopters from a nearby resort of Sochi, hovered overhead to lighten the midnight skies and guide the rescue work. In the glare of the helicopter's searchlights the sea appeared as a film of oil and paint dotted with bodies, barrels, debris and hundreds of people. Some were clinging to life rafts, some had life jackets and most were swimming or treading water. 'Women and children were the first we tried to rescue, said one sailor. 'One father saved his three girls who were terrified, all covered in oil. They seemed unable to realise what was happening to them.'

Later 80 divers attempted to retrieve bodies from the wreckage, nearly 150 feet below the waves. Their work was hampered because a hole in the side of the liner was facing the sea bed and winds were high. Some relatives buried their dead. About 400 other relatives were given information twice a day and survivors were sent home.

One startling aspect sets this tragedy apart from all previous disasters in the Soviet Union. On direct orders from Gorbachev the world was told about it quickly and in detail. The Soviet leader, it seems, wanted to turn the catastrophe into a pure case of how to campaign for more openness, should work. The first word of the accident came 18 hours after it had happened, but later the Soviet media gave extraordinarily detailed coverage and officials organised frequent press conferences. The *Admiral Nakimov* reports however do not mean that openness has no limits. But the Soviet Union's leader recognised that there can be no reform of the country's notorious inefficiency unless there is reform and unless the country faces up to its problems. That means the people must be trusted with more information and the controllers of the information have to learn to break the secret habits of decades.

My superficial acquaintanceship with Russia and its people had made me feel optimistic about prospects of better cooperation in the years ahead.

CANADA – 1973

My second visit to Canada was to the west coast where I stayed with a generous and friendly young medical couple who had trained in Britain, and lived on the outskirts of Vancouver. They lived in a most comfortable beautifully situated wooden house and told me that only the really affluent people lived in stone houses. The mountain ranges to the east and north cut off the cold Arctic air and Vancouver Island to the west protects Vancouver from the rough Pacific winds. The climate is pleasantly mild so that it is possible to swim in the English Bay, warmed by the Japanese currents, yet go up on the cable car to the top of Grouse Mountain 20 minutes away and be among the snow.

When I went up there, I had my cine-camera and saw only one man admiring the view. Determined to take home visual evidence of snow in summertime in Vancouver, I went up to the man hoping that he would take some cine-film of me in the snow.

'Do you speak English?'

'Yes – my name is Naish and I'm a physician from Bristol.'

So I have my small piece of cine-film.

We talked about Vancouver and medicine. He advised me to go to Stanley Park where there is a unique collection of totem poles carved over the centuries by British Columbia's Coast Indians. Also in Stanley Park is the Nine O'Clock Gun, the Vancouver equivalent of Big Ben, which is fired every evening.

However, I was there primarily to learn about medicine. Taking part in a case conference at the Veterans' Hospital, I saw some of the American Indians who certainly have not benefited from contact with the so-called civilised white man. There were cases of tuberculosis, syphilis, alcoholic cirrhosis of the liver, and no doubt now there will be AIDS also.

Vancouver Harbour is spanned by the Lion's Gate Bridge – the longest in the Commonwealth – and I spent some time in the hospital on the other side. A number of the physiotherapists and occupational therapists had been trained in the UK and we had much in common. I had given a BMA lecture at Tavistock Square in London on occupational therapy, illustrated with slides taken in Eastbourne. There is so much colour and activity in departments of occupational therapy anywhere in the world that it is difficult to restrain oneself from being trigger-happy.

Kenneth Vickery, one of the most eminent men in what used to be called the public health service, chose to remain in Eastbourne although he could have taken much more senior posts in major centres.

Kenneth enhanced his reputation for health promotion by persuasive publications and after-dinner advocacy. He talked of the growing needs of the elderly – referring to the HMSO document *The Population of Britain* – and described our rival seaside resort of Folkestone as for the continent, Eastbourne for the incontinent.

At the annual mayoral banquet, presided over by a most charming and competent lady mayoress, he said that she was rather modest – if you pull her chain she flushes.

Many years before the development of the present all-embracing social services organisation, he persuaded the local authority to provide homes for the infirm elderly.

Kenneth and I had a good working relationship, meeting at regular intervals to exchange information about health service plans of the local authority and developments in the hospitals. We had many common interests, including paying respects to our forebears, whose work is often forgotten by the present generation.

When I called to inform him about the recent death of a colleague, he said that he had already been told. When I said, 'Sorry for an unnecessary call,' he replied to my surprise, 'Don't worry. I always like to hear about people dying.'

He and I, in our respective spheres, together with the general practitioners, endured a severe crisis of shortage of hospital facilities for the aged. The hardship was so intense that it was necessary for the local authority to modify its residential places for the elderly infirm and supportive community services whilst awaiting the provision of hospital beds. Meanwhile the residential homes resembled nursing homes with a heavy load of aged sick.

Uniquely for the country, the local authorities (East Sussex and Eastbourne) agreed to assign geriatric health visitors to the geriatric consultant to ensure that those patients with the most need were admitted to the scarce hospital beds.

About that time, Dr C.A. Boucher, adviser to the then Ministry of Health, came to Eastbourne to discuss the 'borderline' between hospital and local authority responsibilities for elderly infirm people. Soon afterwards the ministry issued guidelines to the NHS based on our experiences in Eastbourne.

One of the consequences of the National Health Service is that consultants often choose to work in a pleasant area – like Eastbourne – rather than remain in a London teaching hospital. One of our first consultants appointed after the start of the Health Service was Aubrey Jenkins, who had been a lecturer at the Postgraduate School at Hammersmith working with the late Professor Ian Aird, before he became a consultant orthopaedic surgeon in Eastbourne. When 'Jenks' died suddenly there was widespread distress.

At nearby Hastings, Bobby Irvine, who reminds me in many ways of Lord Hailsham, chose to swim against the tide and develop a geriatric service. Although he might well have been a consultant at Guy's, where he trained, he made an international name by his work, his writings and his personality. Ultimately he was elected president of the British Geriatrics Society.

My impression is that relatively few people in this country realise that Canada is the second largest country in the world, exceeded in size only by the Soviet Union. That it happens to have more lakes than the rest of the world combined is not likely to excite the man in the street.

As a doctor, I knew that Sir William Osler who lived from 1849–1919 was born in Ontario and had had a greater influence on modern medical practice than perhaps any other man. He taught such great doctors as the Mayo brothers, and Harvey Cushing, the neurologist. His book *Aequanimitas* is a masterpiece.

Sir Frederick Banting (1891–1941) was the son of an Ontario farmer and won a Nobel Prize for discovering along with another Canadian, Dr Charles Best, that diabetes is caused by or perhaps more correctly associated with, a lack of insulin.

Wilder Penfield left Canada to work in America and is recognised as the greatest contributor to neurology and neurosurgery in recent times, having exceptional knowledge of epilepsy.

Yet the Canadian doctors I met were modest and unassuming, invariably polite to a nonentity like myself.

When not attending meetings or visiting hospitals I saw something of the Canadian loggers. Just as the ballet in Russia and the opera in Italy had seemed to me to be the world's best, so the Canadian loggers are quite exceptional. We were treated to a display of competitive hand-sawing of logs – they now use electric saws – and axe throwing. They could throw a heavy axe so that it would embed itself in a tree trunk with deadly accuracy.

The BMA president at the time, the late Sir Thomas Holmes-Sellors, a world famous thoracic surgeon, like the president of the Canadian Medical Association, could barely lift the axe. Then the loggers demonstrated how to shin up a tree at amazing speed wearing crampons. All of this I recorded on cine. I also took pictures of the huge rafts of logs coming down river to Vancouver from the lumber camps. The loggers are a tough bunch of men, unequalled by anyone in the rest of the world.

During my stay in Vancouver I was very hospitably entertained by a local doctor, Dr Peter Robson, whose father was one of my colleagues who practised at Herstmonceux in Sussex.

Another unique feature of Canada is the Canadian Mounted Police. As a boy, I had dreams of joining the police, but doubt if I have the necessary physical or psychological qualities required. It is an interesting aspect of travel to observe how police function in different countries. I made many friends in the Eastbourne police 40 years ago, when it was a relatively small county borough force.

One cold November morning, a workman wearing Wellington boots was maintaining a conveyor belt used for sifting shingle on the Crumbles in Eastbourne when his mate started the machinery in error, so that this man had his foot trapped in a large cog wheel at the top of a steel tower. All the practising doctors were out on their rounds, including the police surgeon. So they phoned me at the hospital and I went immediately with a syringe and morphia. At that time I had a fear of heights, but with my friend, a police sergeant, we climbed up a steel ladder, and gave the man a shot of morphia. Then we managed to get his foot out of the machinery. By this time the fire brigade had arrived so we fixed a stretcher to a rope at the tip of their turntable ladder and lowered him to the ground. He was in a fairly shocked state, so I asked a police officer to drive my car so that I could accompany the patient in the ambulance to hospital. As we sped along, I became increasingly concerned about the patient who had remained silent, making no complaint of pain despite his badly injured foot.

It was I who nearly fainted when he spoke for the first time and said, 'Doctor, do you know a good cure for chilblains.'

Fortunately, the end result was good after many weeks in hospital.

So I returned from Canada, as usual glad to be home again.

JAMAICA – APRIL 1974

The fairest island that eyes have beheld, was how Christopher Columbus described Jamaica – and even then, in 1494, he had visited quite a number of other islands, the Canaries, Cuba, Haiti – so that he was well able to make comparisons. My purpose in going there was primarily to enhance my limited medical knowledge, but I learnt a great deal about the history of the island and enjoyed the marvellous climate. The original inhabitants, the Arawak Indians, called it the land of wood and water, Xamayaca, but they were wiped out by the Spaniards who arrived in the sixteenth century. Since 1655, British influence has been predominant, with place names like Bath, Cambridge and Newport. Devon House is a fine old house, now a national museum. The people are dignified and proud of their independence, which began in 1962. No one I met seemed resentful about the treatment the islanders had received from the British pirates or buccaneers. None of them knew that the word 'buccaneer' is derived from '*boucan*', the frame on which early settlers dried meat and pork which they sold to the Spaniards.

To work the sugar plantations, slaves were imported from Africa in increasing numbers so that in 1785 Jamaica had 250,000 slave workers, outnumbering the white population by ten to one. It was not until 1834 that slavery was abolished.

Although sugar is still a major source of wealth, bauxite, the precursor of aluminium, is produced in large quantities both in Jamaica and in Guyana.

As a venue for a medical meeting, the West Indies has much to recommend it. My companion on the flight out was the then editor of *World Medicine*, Dr Michael O'Donnell, who had chosen journalism rather than medical practice. There are many precedents for doing so – including Somerset Maugham. A few years ago, I attended a most interesting meeting at the Royal Society of Medicine when David Owen, Jonathan Miller and Miriam Stoppard explained why they had opted for a career other than clinical medicine. All had the advantage of being well above average in intelligence and so were capable of succeeding in other fields. It would not have been realistic to apply the old jibe levelled at medical administrators as being failed clinicians.

The organisers had compiled a most interesting programme and the principal guest speaker was Dr Debakey, the world-famous heart surgeon. His participation was sponsored by one of the major international pharmaceutical firms who arranged his flight from Houston. This firm, like others, had a hospitality room which by chance was being managed by an English executive whom I had met some years earlier when he was a medical representative. He invited me to have a drink after Dr Debakey's lecture, at which I sat in the rear row of seats. So I was first out and arrived simultaneously in the hospitality room with Dr Debakey. Like all eminent men I have been privileged to meet, he talked to me like an equal and asked searching questions about the functions of the British National Health Service.

There was ample time for leisure as well as for participating in the scientific meetings. The trade winds prevent the sun from being uncomfortably hot, but led some of my colleagues to overdo exposure to sunlight and suffer from sunburn. A cup of strong Blue Mountain coffee with a glass of Tia Maria was a favourite drink to sip under a beach umbrella.

One of the local hospital consultants told me how the infamous Welshman Henry Morgan, who was tried for piracy in London, was later knighted and returned to

Jamaica as governor. When he died in 1688, he was given a state funeral. He also told me that Jamaica's national bird is the Doctor Bird – and unashamedly said that it has a typically Jamaican sense of the dramatic and likes to show off.

Near Kingston is Port Royal, once the wickedest and most debauched city in the New World. Perhaps providentially, on 7th June, 1692, two thirds of the town sank under the sea in a violent earthquake followed by a tidal wave.

There is worldwide interest in the museum housed in the former Naval Hospital, built in 1819, to deal with yellow fever. The harbour near Port Royal is one of the richest archaeological sites in the world – however I had come to study the medical services and missed out on so many of the fascinating aspects of life in Jamaica, even though we were received with great kindness and offered generous hospitality, extending to lessons in limbo dancing. 'Howdy and tenky no bruck no square' means, 'How do you do, and thank you break no bones', that is to say, 'It is not only good manners to be polite, but it does no harm.'

MAJORCA – 1975

The participants in the visit to the USSR in 1972 very generously made a collection on the plane during the return journey to express their thanks to me for organising the trip. With the money collected I bought a cine-camera and made a documentary film about geriatric work in Eastbourne. When I was asked to show the film to the annual meeting of the Spanish Medical Association in Majorca in 1975, I expected that most of the Spanish doctors would speak English. To my surprise, this was not the case, so that I had to do the commentary in Italian because my knowledge of Spanish was poor. It was therefore rather generous of the local paper to publish the following article:

Majorca Daily Bulletin Wednesday 7th May, 1975

BRITISH APPROACH TO GERONTOLOGY
The British contribution to the Eighth National Congress of Gerontology has been considerable, beginning with Professor Brocklehurst of the University of Manchester, whose work in the field of geriatric medicine is most notable.
Another of the British doctors is Dr I. M. Brown of Eastbourne, who projected a very significant film entitled *Team Work on the Costa Geriatrica*. He is at the Hotel Victoria.
The *Costa Geriatrica*, as I discovered, is an area where there are 30 per cent of the population aged 65 and over, the highest in the world.
The film, which was in colour, showed a number of very enlightening views of the standard British approach to geriatrics all in very modern and congenial

surroundings of Southern England in the Downs area of Sussex.

Some of the scenes, with fantastic attention to the medical detail, were most revealing of the British approach to geriatrics, which studies and sets in motion a most complete organisation, and with a team work which involved everyone connected with it.

'Unless everyone is working together as a team,' Dr Brown explained, 'you cannot have a really efficient organisation.'

How would you express the British approach to gerontology?

'I would say, the same standards of care for old people as for people at any other age. As a matter of fact, the British concern for the medical care of the aged probably leads the world.'

And in rejuvenation?

'I would say that it is fundamentally difficult to reverse the ageing process. But what we try to do is to give the best possible treatment to the aged, as you would to a child or an adult or any working individual.'

How did the *Costa Geriatrica* come into existence?

'Because in England every year, 1,000 people retire to Eastbourne, mostly from London. In a survey I made, only one patient in five in the geriatric wards were recorded as being born locally.

'At the last international congress of gerontology in Kiev, USSR, attention was drawn to the problems caused by large-scale migration of elderly retired persons to the South Coast of England.

'This is very different from most countries, where the elderly retired usually remain in the same area where they have been living previously.

'As far as the British approach to geriatrics is concerned, the textbook of Professor J.C. Brocklehurst is, I would say, the most authoritative and comprehensive up-to-date publication in the world.

Apart from the scientific aspects of the meeting, I was able to see a little of this beautiful island, the largest and most important of the Balearic Islands. They constitute one of the 50 provinces of Spain and are as much a part of Spain as Wales is of the United Kingdom.

Majorca is of course a very popular package holiday resort for Britons, the great majority of whom behave reasonably. A few of those who did not were unaware why they had to return to England by stretcher.

Four-fifths of the Balearic islanders, who total about 500,000, live in Majorca, and a high percentage are involved in the tourist industry.

They are jolly and hospitable if treated in a decent way and few seem to be aware that men lived on the island as far back as 4,000 BC. Nor were they especially interested in the fact that, in the distant past, the dead were buried sitting on their heels, sometimes being later cremated – strange in a Catholic country, although Catholicism had not yet begun to influence their customs. Like our Martello Towers on the south coast of England – the name is derived from Mortella Point in Corsica – the Majorcans have *tayalots* (watchtowers).

Moorish influence is still in evidence – irrigation systems, land terracing, the Arab chain pump (*noria*) and windmills.

If you go to Majorca, enjoy the sun.

JAPAN – 1979–80

In December 1979, after retiring from hospital, we went to Japan to visit our daughter Rosalind. She had been teaching English in Paris when she learnt that the Japanese Government wanted about 30 teachers of English to work in Japan. After an interview at the Japanese Embassy in London she was selected as one of the group.

En route to Japan, a list of Japanese educational establishments were circulated in the plane, with places at schools, polytechnics and universities. Rosalind had the good fortune to be allocated to Gakushuin University in Tokyo – the Oxford and Cambridge of Japan – where the senior professor in the department of English, Professor Usami, was tutor to the son of the emperor. A very prestigious establishment, as we later discovered.

The journey from Heathrow was with Japanese Air Lines and we were cosseted by courteous and attentive stewardesses. Slippers were provided for each passenger and warm face flannels were offered so that one could relax comfortably. Then a small porcelain beaker with warm saké was offered to us all with in-flight movies, as is customary in other long-haul airlines.

Our staging point was Anchorage, Alaska, a bleak environment with a warm hospitable airport lounge. There was time to take a few photographs before we continued the journey in the plane which had been spotlessly cleaned during the brief halt.

Japanese Air Lines had provided me with a pack of visiting cards, with English on one side and Japanese on the other. These were to prove most useful.

Rosalind was waiting for us at the Shiba Hotel although we arrived quite late by Tokyo time, and we had a brief exchange of experiences before she returned to her flat on the university campus. Tokyo is a safe city for young women at night – quite unlike London.

We had studied various books about Japan – how they had developed as a nation, how they behaved during the war, the fascinating book about Pearl Harbor – *At Dawn We Slept* by Gordon Prange, with its account of the brilliant action of the Japanese fleet and air force and the inadequacy of the American defences. Everyone should read the *American Caesar* by William Manchester about General Douglas McArthur, probably the most brilliant general of the last war. He had so many abnormal facets in his character that I for one was astounded by what I read. Virtually all the war leaders, however brilliant, had abnormal traits which were not disclosed during hostilities. We were repeatedly reminded of the villainy of the mass murderer Josef Stalin and of the paranoia of Adolf Hitler, but both had exceptional qualities and both were able to control their generals as well as the common man. Even Benito Mussolini, in spite of his buffoonery, had outstanding gifts.

Japan had benefited greatly from the McArthur era and even now has marked traditional attitudes in a modern highly sophisticated society. As in many other countries, religion is less dominant than formerly. There has been a drift away from the country to the city – less than seven per cent of the population now depend on agriculture for more than half their income. More than half the total population of Japan now lives in cities with populations of 100,000 or more.

There is considerable loyalty to the employing organisation, which will provide educational and sports facilities, health care, housing and various perquisites. In the countryside, after the Second World War the Occupation authorities saw the domination of rural society by the landlord class as one of the major obstacles to the democratisation of Japanese society and so transferred ownership of land from landlord to tenant.

In the cities industrial organisations are truly family enterprises. The Japanese worker often spends time when away from work on such activities as fishing with workmates, rather than at home, as is the case in most other countries. He may be regarded as more interested in his work than his family, but everyone I spoke to seemed quite happy with this way of life.

At work, the entire staff wear the same uniform, with no class distinction, the only difference between the employees being in their seniority and degree of intelligence and industry – a meritocracy. The system works extremely well and where industry in Great Britain is run on the same lines it seems to be successful. We still have, however, some management which is unwilling or incapable of progress. And too many of our workers are of similar attitude, with many, like some of their managers, unable to grasp the essentials of industrial relations which lead to success.

We were able to identify Japanese executives by their custom of wearing white shirts, apparently an essential part of the business executives' dress. So in a train, one would approach an executive, produce the bilingual visiting card and he would do likewise. He probably spoke a little English and could advise us which station would be near the university. All we could say then was, 'Thank you,' *'Dom arigato'*.

I had joined the Japan Society of London before retiring and learnt a little about their general philosophy, witnessed a tea ceremony and attended their annual dinner in London, honoured then by the presence of the ambassador and his wife, Mr and Mrs Fujiyama. We were pleased to read that Lord Carrington, when Secretary of State for Foreign and Commonwealth Affairs, gave a farewell luncheon on 6th January 1982 at Admiralty House in honour of Mr and Mrs Fujiyama.

After we had visited Rosalind in her office at the University, we were taken by her and a friend, Keiko, to visit a Shinto temple. The approaches were thronged by Japanese coming to pay their respects and seek help in some cases. The procedure adopted by the supplicant was to draw the attention of the gods to their presence by clapping hands or ringing a small bell.

Nearby there was incense burning. We were told that by passing one's hand through the smoke and then rubbing aches and pains there would be a beneficial response. It so happened that I had a painful shoulder at the time, but the discomfort did not entirely disappear when I tried the remedy. From Tokyo we went by train to nearby Kamakura to see the famous figure of the great Buddha – Daibutsu Kamakura. A huge gilt bronze statue built in the thirteenth century, it is invariably in tourist itineraries and we found it fascinating, so that we still have a plaster cast model at home. We thought it superb (*migoto*) and really monumental (*dodotarumono*).

From Tokyo one can take the bullet train – the *Shinkansen* – to Kyoto, also on the mainland, that is on the island of Honshu. (Unfortunately we were unable to visit Hokkaido, the northern island, or Shikoku or Kyushu in the south.)

Dominating the city of Tokyo is Mount Fuji, with its snow-capped summit. Fuji is venerated by the Japanese and a visit there in cherry blossom time is an unforgettable experience.

We would have liked to stay at a Japanese-style inn – a *ryokan*, with old-style furnishing. There, breakfast is usually a bowl of rice, soya bean soup, seaweed and raw eggs. Choosing food in Japanese restaurants is made easy because many have plastic models of their special dishes and it is necessary only to point to one's choice. Seafood specialities such as *sushi*, *sashini* and *tempura* were my favourites – *tempura* is fresh fish – horse mackerel, cuttlefish, conger eel, river trout and whitebait. In a Japanese-style, as opposed to a Western-style restaurant, it is customary to take off one's shoes at the door. Also, it is usual to sit on the floor, which I personally found uncomfortable.

We visited what was then the tallest building in Tokyo – called Sunshine City. On the flat roof was an ingenious series of water jets or miniature fountains, which spelt out the English word 'Welcome'. Unfortunately, it was not possible to get a good view of the city because the top was shrouded in mist. As I had had a similar experience at the top of the *Tour Montparnasse* in Paris, it was not altogether surprising.

We were sorry to leave Japan, but excited at the prospect of seeing Hong Kong for the first time. By a stroke of good fortune, I had met a Miss Jill Fox when she was visiting Eastbourne to see her uncle, a patient under my care in St Mary's Hospital. After I discussed her uncle's case she explained that she was on the civilian staff of the Hong Kong police and would be pleased to show us the sights of Hong Kong if ever we were to go there. I said that this was highly unlikely, but within a year we were being greeted by her at Hong Kong airport.

The city is well known throughout the world from film and television productions even if one has not had the good fortune to visit the area.

A panoramic view of the harbour can be obtained from the Peak district, where we were taken for dinner shortly after arrival. Next day we visited Repulse Bay, with a flavour of the Victorian era, then went by the Star Ferry to Aberdeen where thousands of local people live in junks, many luxuriously furnished, with television and all kinds of modern amenities. I decided to get a suit made and went to a tailor called Sam who quickly measured me and had the suit handmade overnight. Dinner on our second night was on a junk in the harbour, and again I felt impelled to take still and cine photographs.

Too soon, we were on our way to Bangkok, with its gilt royal palace and many canals – Klongs – some of which have been filled in to provide roads for the rapidly increasing traffic.

However, we did go on a flat-bottomed boat on a Klong to the well-known Floating Market where traders, selling mainly fruit and vegetables, live in junks cooking on charcoal stoves. A spectacle available for the tourist is a fight between a snake and a mongoose – this I was able to record on cine-film. On this particular occasion the mongoose killed the snake.

Thailand has its own fascination with a great deal of historical interest and beautiful beaches such as Pattaya, where we spent a few days.

The visit was much too short and we still recall the people and the country with affection, although I had had preconceived ideas based on the appalling cruelty meted out to British prisoners of war.

But on reflection I realise that no army selects its élite to staff prisoner of war camps. Every POW has memories of some good aspects of life in a prison camp. My own experience was that British camps were not invariably without their imperfections.

We still correspond with friends in Japan and have had Japanese guests stay with us in Eastbourne.

We may have been fortunate, but our impressions of Japan and the Japanese people were certainly favourable.

A LIGHTNING TOUR OF EUROPE

with Japanese friends

My younger daughter Rosalind became friendly with a Japanese lady called Junko, whose husband held a senior medical administrative position in Tokyo. Like so many of the Japanese people I met, she was friendly, courteous, and invariably helpful. My only concept of Japanese before 1980 was obtained from colleagues who had been prisoners of war.

Junko was so kind to Rosalind that we invited her to join us on a family holiday in Brittany where we had a villa near Trégastel, with nine in our family group.

Junko enjoyed her stay and used to go regularly to the local post office to telephone her husband in Tokyo, so that finally he decided to come to Europe to see some of the countries for himself.

He started by inviting Rosalind to fly with Junko from nearby Morlaix airport to London where they met at the Hilton Hotel. Then on to the superb Excelsior Hotel on the Via Veneto in Rome where I had stayed for a week in 1944, when it was an officers' leave centre. With a Japanese guide who could speak English, French and Italian, they managed to visit the Colosseum, the Pantheon, Piazza Navona, Piazza del Popolo and, of course, St Peter's. But it takes years, not days, to form an impression of Rome.

Then on to the Villa d'Este at Cernobbio, at the southern end of Lake Como. This magnificent hotel was a Cardinal's Palace in the sixteenth century, but after the briefest stay they took the railway to the Jungfraujoch, had a Japanese meal in the restaurant at 11,000 feet and admired the magnificent views. Rosalind was given the chance of driving down in the Mercedes – she said that it was like driving a double bed.

She seemed to remember the smoked trout with whipped cream at the Hotel Baur on Lake Zurich more than the scenery – it was quite misty.

By the next day they were staying in the Hotel Vier Jahreszeiten in Hamburg, which Rosalind thought was a beautiful city, but less attractive than Frankfurt, although she liked Heidelberg. The Vier Jahreszeiten won an award for being the best hotel in Germany, very spacious, with marvellous tapestries and beautiful old furniture.

Then to Copenhagen where Rosalind had been as a child, followed by a stay in the Ritz in Paris, where Rosalind felt that she could take the initiative and show her Japanese friends around, before they returned to Japan.

We had dinner in the main Japanese restaurant a year or so later, after a somewhat hair-raising drive from the suburbs (Asnières), and round the Arc de Triomphe at night – the French version of Hyde Park Corner – but more difficult for the driver with a GB plate who seems to be a fair target for the leather-suited young French motor cyclists who zoomed around our car at breakneck speed.

The Japanese were very receptive and quickly grasped the main differences between the various European countries in spite of such an extremely brief stay.

Scenically, of course, nothing could compare with Mount Fuji. It was impossible for them to grasp the political differences, but our MP, Mr Ian Gow, had given an interview to Rosalind before she went to Japan, so that the British political system was taped and played back to all the students of English at Gakushuin University.

She was extremely fortunate in having such a grand tour of Europe and we still have visitors from Japan who have been told something of the British way of life.

CHRISTMAS IN ROME – DECEMBER 1984

Rome, the Eternal City, became world famous as the capital of the Roman Empire, the focal point of western Christendom and the Roman Catholic church, and one of the great artistic centres of the world. Yet it became the capital of the Republic of Italy on its creation only just over a hundred years ago in 1862.

The foundation of Rome is said to date from 753 BC and as it became more powerful successive emperors erected larger and more handsome public buildings, temples, roads and aqueducts. Each emperor vied with his predecessors in altering and embellishing the city with victory columns, triumphal arches, theatres and mausoleums.

Evidence of Rome becoming the spiritual centre of Christendom remains in the shape of large basilicas founded in the fourth and fifth century. The four patriarchal basilicas – that is, those of which the Pope is priest – are St Peter's, St John Lateran, St Maria Maggiore and St Paul's, outside the walls.

Christmas in Rome is celebrated as an important religious festival, with relatively less of the vulgar commercial trappings which are so obvious in other western capital cities. Dry, sunny weather, with the temperature slightly above that prevailing in the south of England in December, is deal for sightseeing. From a small hotel near the main railway station (Termini) it is possible to visit most of the interesting parts of the old city on foot.

Public transport – mainly buses – is inexpensive for any length of journey. Tickets can be purchased from transport kiosks or tobacconists, and most buses have ticket-cancelling machines, so have no bus conductors.

One particularly worthwhile trip can be done on a No. 30 tram. From Piazza Risorgimento, near St Peter's, it crosses the River Tiber, skirts the Borghese Gardens and passes quite a number of interesting buildings, circling the old town.

In common with all major cities, Rome is experiencing increasing traffic congestion, with drivers showing less respect for traffic lights than is the case in England. It is unwise to assume that one can cross on a light-controlled pedestrian crossing with safety.

Unlike our cities, Rome appears to have no level or multi-storey car parks, and most streets have cars parked on both sides. It looks as if some cars have been parked there for weeks or possibly months. When traffic congestion becomes particularly acute, every driver seems to believe that the solution is to be found by repeated sounding of the car horn. Not surprisingly, a fairly large number of cars have dents and scrapes on the bodywork.

One of the unusual features of Rome is that street lighting is much less effective than in other capital cities.

From Termini the Colosseum is reached easily on foot. It is the largest structure left by Roman antiquity and has provided the model for sports arenas right down to modern times. So named because it was built on the site of a colossal statue of Nero, it could accommodate 50,000 spectators. Originally covered by a vast awning supported by masts, it had, underneath the arena, changing rooms for 1,000 gladiators and cages for 5,000 wild beasts.

Unfortunately, the building has suffered greatly from earthquakes, fires, neglect and dilapidation. To make matters worse, marble and brick has been pilfered to build palaces elsewhere. But it remains as a fascinating relic of the great Roman empire.

Quite near the Colosseum is the church of San Pietro in Vincoli – St Peter in Chains. The relics – chains which

Peter was traditionally believed to have worn in the Mamertine Prison, lie in a glass case on the high altar. This church, one of the oldest in Rome, contains the finest achievements in sculpture in the world, such as the *Moses* by Michaelangelo. Its massive dominance, perfect symmetry and impression of vitality have a profound effect even on the uninitiated like myself. A beautifully created Christmas crib was a temporary addition to the church interior.

Within sight of the Colosseum is the National Monument to Victor Emmanuel II, the largest and most magnificent monument in Italy, built in white Brescia marble. Behind is the Capitol, the smallest but historically the most important of Rome's seven hills. Adjacent, approached by a flight of 122 steps, is the church of Santa Maria in Aracoeli (that means on the altar of heaven). Here again was an outstanding Christmas crib. In the north aisle is a carved wooden image of the infant Christ (*Santo Bambino*) which is the subject of particular veneration at Christmas.

The remains of the Roman forum lie between the Capitol and the Colosseum. Destruction of the forum began in the sixth century and the ruins were uncovered only 100 years ago.

To help the visitor to identify and appreciate the innumerable monuments, churches, museums, temples, formations and gardens there are dozens of published guides printed in just about every language of the world. In my opinion, no other capital city has such a vast diversity of interest for the tourist.

Most visitors gravitate, soon after arriving in Rome, to St Peter's and the Vatican. It is a unique experience to see and hear the Pope address a huge crowd in St Peter's Square, with television relaying his message around the world. The present Polish Pope, John Paul II, the supreme head of the Roman Catholic Church, with 700,000,000 adherents, is the first non-Italian to be selected for this high office for many years. At the conclusion of each address he adds a few words of greeting in many different languages, receiving recognition from pilgrims in the vast assembly gathered from all over the world, who clap and cheer as they recognise their mother tongue.

The Vatican Museum contain one of the world's greatest art collections. There, the visitor can profitably spend hours in the Sistine Chapel admiring the incredibly beautiful murals and frescoes by Michaelangelo and other great masters.

St Peter's is on the other side of the River Tiber from the old town. Nearby is the area of Trastevere (*Trans Tiberum* – Across the Tiber), with its narrow streets, old houses, open-air markets and numerous small restaurants or *trattoria*. Visitors are advised to explore Trastevere, especially to find inexpensive meals in family-run establishments. Amongst popular Roman dishes are *stracciatella*, meat broth containing eggs, semolina, Parmesan cheese and parsley – *saltimbocca*, stuffed veal cutlets – and *trippa alla Romana* – strips of tripe cooked with onions, carrots, mint leaves and Parmesan cheese.

It seemed to me that fewer Italians than formerly drink wine with meals, many, especially the young, preferring *aqua minerale* (mineral water). But cigarette smoking seems to be more prevalent than in England, where it is steadily declining especially in the managerial and professional groups.

Like all capital cities, Rome has a higher percentage of immigrants than the country as a whole. But the prevailing impression of a unique city populated by friendly, cheerful, articulate Roman citizenry proud of their fine heritage.

FRANCE

How do you begin to talk about a country you have been visiting regularly for more than fifty years?
You cannot do better than start in Paris at the Place de la Concorde. It was designed by Gabriel in 1753 at the command of the King and for this reason was initially called Place Louis XV. At the time of the French revolution, it was the site of the scaffold. So it has witnessed both festivities and executions.

On a mild spring evening, with the fountains floodlit, nothing can compare with the view up the Champs Elysées towards the Arc de Triomphe, the church of the Madeleine on the right and the River Seine on the left.

At the International Hospital Federation Congress in Paris in 1963 our hosts did everything possible to make us feel welcome, and show us the best that Paris has to offer. The vista from the top of the Eiffel Tower is marvellous. We had a river trip on the Seine on a *bateau mouche* and dinner at the Palace of Versailles. We were the first international organisation to be allowed to dine there in lounge suits out of deference to the Americans who could not easily bring a white tie and tails in one small flight bag.

Our buses assembled at the Place de la Concorde, in the early evening, marshalled by the redoubtable Monsieur Faucon, a mixture of doctor, administrator and regimental sergeant major. Unfortunately, the driver of the chartered bus in which I travelled did not know the way to Versailles, which I found quite extraordinary. He was not an intellectual and had difficulty in starting the bus, so was unable to follow the one in front. The bus was well-oiled, as was the driver.

Fortunately I was able to guide him to Versailles.

We arrived in daylight and could see why the chateau is

justly described as being among the most beautiful, famous and historical sights in Europe.

The architecture, interior, park and in fact, the entire court of the French Kings at Versailles in the seventeenth and eighteenth century served as a model for many European royal and princely courts of that time.

We had a magnificent dinner in the Hall of Mirrors, but as had happened in Venice a couple of years before, the after-dinner speeches were not only too long but were translated following each speech into several languages. As a result, quite a number of those present engaged in a lively and, at times, noisy argumentative conversation nearly as bad as our House of Commons.

After a reception at the *Hotel de Ville* (the Town Hall) on the following evening, we walked down to the Seine, passed Notre Dame and then along the south bank to the Hôpital Pitiè-Salpetrière. This is the Paris equivalent of St Mary's Hospital in Eastbourne – an old institution, very much bigger of course, but with a similar atmosphere. When we had had another glass of wine with the hospital staff everyone started to drift back to their hotels. We were bade *adieu* by magnificently dressed hospital porters at the front door. With their white ties and tails, gold chains and war medals, they looked more magnificent than any of the notabilities from Paris or the rest of the world. Once again, I could not resist taking a photograph of them at the main entrance.

Instead of accompanying my colleagues back to their hotels, I re-entered the Salpetrière and walked round the wards talking to the patients. No one questioned my presence.

Not long before our meeting in Paris, a man dressed in a white coat walked round the wards of a hospital in Leeds. He asked a number of patients if he could check their pulse rate, apologised for not having a watch, and was 'lent' one by quite a number of patients. Shortly afterwards he left the hospital with a pocketful of wristwatches and was never seen again.

After going round the wards, I decided to visit the hospital kitchens to see for myself how the famed French cuisine was prepared for the patients. Admittedly this was in 1963, but I was not particularly impressed. There was only one man in the vast kitchen, a German, hopelessly drunk. He thought that I was a German and offered to show me how sacks of potatoes were tipped into cauldrons, to prepare soup. Although he managed to hoist the sack on to his broad shoulders, he was what we English would call 'legless' and fell to the ground with the potato sack on top of his inert body. So I propped him up against the cauldron, ensured that he was breathing, and left.

Dr W. A. J. Farndale, Ph.D., Dr J.S. Cayla, *Directeur de l'Ecole Nationale de la Santé Publique* and our Professor T.E. Chester, Professor of Social Administration at Manchester University, have written an excellent book on French Hospitals and Medical Care Services.

Dr Farndale kindly invited me to lecture on European Health Services at the Polytechnic of the South Bank in London, although he knows far more about the subject than I do.

At the time of our visit, more than half the hospital beds in France were in public hospitals, the remainder being in various clinics and private hospitals.

We also visited the modern St Nazaire Hospital built in 1960 with about 500 beds, the large Cochin Hospital with nearly 2,000 beds, built in 1780, but now modernised and very impressive. It is in the Montparnasse area and has a fine reputation for accident surgery, like our Birmingham Accident Hospital.

We formed the impression that there were fewer staff in French hospitals – certainly in 1987 there is a good deal of over-staffing in British hospitals. Our DHSS is well aware of this and is actively dealing with the matter – not a popular task.

Each ward has a *garçon*, who seemed to be a most invaluable member of the staff. He was a versatile and resourceful 'Jack of All Trades'. I had a lengthy conversation with a *garçon* at the Hôpital Broussais. Although the organisation may be different now, the pharmacy dealt not only with the medicines, but also haematology (blood examination) and blood transfusion services.

Naturally there have been many changes in the system of running French hospitals during the past 25 years. Then, there was no organised out-patient appointment system. One of the paradoxes of our system now is that on a fair number of occasions, the patient does not turn up for the out-patient appointment given, so that I used to have to fill in time waiting for the next patient to arrive.

Our standard of general practice is now excellent. Some doctors send lengthy typewritten letters of referral. Others write in long hand.

When I was doing a ward round, I was handed the case notes of a patient marked 'ONION'.

'Good morning, Mr Onion,' said I, in my best bedside manner, 'And how are you today?'

'Sir,' said the staff nurse, 'his name is O'nion, not Onion.'

'How do you know?'

'Well,' she said, 'if you look at the doctor's referral letter you will see that he has put a suppository between the O and the N.'

I have learned a great deal from French hospitals. Many years ago, when going on holiday to Brittany with my wife and two small children, we were crossing from Newhaven to Dieppe in fairly rough weather. My wife took the two girls to the ladies' sleeping accommodation and I went off to the bunks for *Messieurs*. In one hand I had my overnight bag, and in the other a satchel with tickets, maps, brochures etc. As I went down the stairway not holding the rails, I pitched forward and sustained a fractured skull.

After admission to the District General Hospital in Dieppe, I received first-class treatment, but noticed a few differences between the then current procedure in French and English hospitals. The first difference I noted was that relatives brought masses of food into the ward for the patients to eat, although it seemed to me that the hospital diet was quite good.

Then there was only one loo for 30 patients and if you have a fractured skull you do not feel like queueing up. As still prevails, the smart young thing on the Continent wears dark glasses. My night nurse was one of them and used to have great difficulty in stumbling round my bed in the dark wearing sunglasses.

However, within a week I was up and persuaded the surgeon to allow me to watch him remove a gall bladder, little knowing that I was to have the same operation more than 45 years later.

Most of my later visits to France were for holidays. We did ultimately get to Benodet in Brittany. This pretty seaside resort is at the mouth of the river Odet as the name implies. It is possible to have a boat trip up to Quimper, an interesting country town with good road access to all the resorts along the coast. It has a reputation for its fine pottery and we still have some which have survived breakage for many years.

The people are very akin to the Cornish folk, have a language of their own and have beautiful distinctive head dresses called *coiffes*. These are frequently worn with a great starched lace collar.

Like the Jews, the Welsh, Irish, Scots and Majorcans, the

Bretons dissipate their energies in trying to maintain the old Celtic language. There is even a Chair of Celtic Language at the University of Rennes, and an association called UDB (Union for the Defence of the Breton Language).

They are fighting a losing battle. The young people I spoke to invariably considered that they would benefit more by spending time learning English rather than Breton.

It is fascinating to see a Breton *pardon*, a manifestation of religious fervour. We were fortunate in being in Brittany during the second half of August and saw the Grand Pardon at St Anne-le-Palud. In the afternoon, candles, banners and statues of saints are carried by men and girls in procession down the hillside to the church. There the faithful seek forgiveness for their sins, fulfil a vow or beg for grace.

Later, there follow festivities, with wrestling – a traditional sport of Breton peasants – dancing the gavotte accompanied by a form of bagpipe called a *biniou*. The refreshments are usually *crêpes* and cider.

But, as happens throughout the world, many of the young prefer discos, and the old customs are at risk.

When I was in Torre del Greco, south of Naples, I was hurrying to catch a suburban train when I found myself in the midst of a religious procession, mainly consisting of older women and a few young girls carrying banners.

To my surprise, a very old man said to me in the local dialect, 'How nice it is to see a young man taking such an active part in our religious festival. None of our young men will do so now, as I did when I was a youth 70 years ago.'

PARIS

Victor Hugo, the greatest French poet of the 19th century, said,

'Cities are bibles of stone. Paris possesses no single dome, roof or pavement which does not convey some message of alliance and of union, and which does not offer some lesson, example, or advice. Let the people of all the world come to this prodigious alphabet of monuments, of tombs and of trophies to learn peace and to unlearn the meaning of hatred. Let them be confident, for Paris has proven itself. To have once been Lutece – in Caesar's time, the oldest part of Paris on the *Ile de la Cité* was occupied by a fortified Gallic settlement, Lutetia Parisiorum – and to have become Paris, what could be a more magnificent symbol! To have been mud and to have become spirit!'

Very few Parisians know that the architect of the Arc de Triomphe was called J.F. Chalgrin, and we were recommended to a small hotel – the Residence Chalgrin in the Rue Chalgrin. It was only a few hundred yards from the Etoile, where stands the Arc de Triomphe, dedicated to the glory of the victorious French armies of the Revolution and of the First Empire. Napoleon ordered the building of the arch in 1806, but did not live to see its completion in 1836. It was in 1920 that the Tomb of the Unknown Soldier, with its perpetual flame was placed there.

It is well worth while taking the lift to the viewing platform to see the panorama, with the twelve avenues converging on the Place de l'Etoile – now called Place Charles de Gaulle. There is the dead straight line of the Champs Elysées going down to the Concorde and to the

Louvre, illuminated at night by hundreds of cars. On the opposite side, in the distance, are the post-war tower blocks of La Défense, Montmartre with the Sacré-Coeur to the north-east, floodlit at night; the Eiffel Tower; the Dome of the Invalides and the Montparnasse Tower. Admittedly the view from the top of the Eiffel Tower is magnificent – it is about six times the height of the Arc de Triomphe, which is 164 feet high. The third tall structure – the *Tour Montparnasse* – is 656 feet high, more than half the height of the Eiffel Tower, but it was shrouded in mist when I went there, so I did not see very much.

There is so much to see and do in Paris that it would be possible to write volumes on the subject. Indeed there are innumerable books about Paris covering every conceivable aspect.

None of the books refer to Mitterand's grand designs on Paris. In the early 1870s as Paris recovered from the horrors of the Commune, a project was launched to build a patriotic monument on the site of the Tuileries Palace (which had been burned by the Communards). It was suggested that a pyramid be erected closing the view westwards of the Cour Napoléon of the Louvre. This project, made of steel and reflecting glass, designed by the Chinese American architect I. M. Pei is now complete. There is already a magnificent new Musée d'Orsay in the old railway station in which I took a number of photographs. The former station makes a first class museum. Mitterand declares, 'I feel like an emperor or architect. I resolve, I decide, I arbitrate.' The old market, Les Halles, like London's Covent Garden, is now occupied by fashionable shops and restaurants. The Centre Pompidou – called the Beaubourg – looks like a petro-chemical refinery from the outside, but houses avant-garde film theatres, art galleries, libraries and a roof-top restaurant where one can have really good inexpensive meals.

At La Villette, in the suburbs, the former abattoir and market site is to be the site of the Tête de Défense arch, designed by the Danish architect Johan-Otto von Spreckelsen, 350 feet high, more than twice the height of the Arc de Triomphe.

If you were to visit Paris, would you seriously consider spending a few hours in a cemetery? For my part I really enjoyed a visit to the largest and finest cemetery – Cimitière du Père-Lachaise, named after the Father Confessor of Louis XIV. It lies north of the Gare de Lyon, has its own metro station, so is quite easy to get to – whether you are dead or alive. All the best people are buried here – Molière, La Fontaine, Balzac, Marcel Proust, Oscar Wilde, Bizet, Dr Guillotin (who invented the guillotine), Edith Piaf – and there is a special dogs' cemetery.

Cremation has taken much of the fascination from such burial grounds.

Especially in springtime, it is most enjoyable to stroll along the leafy boulevards. Baron Georges-Eugene Haussmann was responsible for extensive rebuilding in Paris under Napoleon III during the latter half of the nineteenth century. The Boulevard Haussman which perpetuates his name was constructed in 1857 and he laid out the Boul' Mich' (the Boulevard St Michel) which is the main thoroughfare in the Latin Quarter and which has many cafés frequented by students.

Much of this might have been destroyed during the last war, but Paris was spared on the authority of General Von Sholtitz, against Hitler's orders.

The cafés are lively animated meeting places and some serve excellent food. Try *quennelles de brochet* – made from river fish, flaked and mixed with breadcrumbs, kidney fat, and eggs, all covered with a sauce made with mushrooms and cream. Of course you must resume your orange juice and lettuce sandwich when you return home.

You may indulge for once in oysters – *fines de Claires*. Epicures prefer the more subtle *belons* and *marennes* and call the *Claire* or *Portugaise* the working man's oyster.

Now walk down the Boul Mich, past the bookshops, down to the river and see the Cathédrale de Nôtre Dame. It was begun in 1163, on the *Ile de la Cité*, and took 150 years to build. Just as I shamelessly copied what I considered to be good features in other hospitals in this country and abroad, recommending their use in Eastbourne, so the builders of Nôtre Dame copied Chartres, Reims, and Amiens.

The view from the 230 foot tower is in many ways more interesting than that from the *Tour d'Eiffel* or *Arc de Triomphe*.

The *Hotel de Ville*, Louvre, Sorbonne and Panthéon are quite near, and their details can be seen easily. The large rose window in the north transept is magnificent, and has about 80 illustrations from the Old Testament. My own experience of photography is limited, so I would not attempt to photograph the rose window. Better get a diapositive taken by a professional if you wish to keep a visual record.

A boat trip from the Pont Neuf is a relatively inexpensive way of seeing so many of the buildings on the river which you may not have time to visit. Down river past the Louvre on the right, the new Musée d'Orsay in the old Gare d'Orsay on the left, under the bridges, Alexandre III, Pont de l'Alma, then past the Eiffel Tower on the left and the Palais de Chaillot on the right. Then the boat will turn round at the Pont Bir Hakeim.

When you return to the Pont Neuf, take a stroll down the Left Bank, past the stalls with prints and books, to Alexander III bridge, turn left, and within a few minutes you will be at the Musée Rodin. Auguste Rodin the sculptor, lived in the former Hôtel Biron, built in 1730, until his death in 1917. If you must be selective because time is pressing, make a point of seeing the full-size copies of the Thinker (*Le Penseur*), The Burghers of Calais, and his 39 studies of Balzac, who said that Paris was a jungle of rapacity, betrayal, greed, ambition and intrigue. Victor Hugo was another of his subjects.

It needs days or even months to see the treasures of the Louvre. A former royal palace, it has been used as a museum since 1793. Every visitor gravitates to the Mona Lisa, but there are masses of interesting paintings, sculptures – including the Venus de Milo – Greek ceramics and crown jewels.

Try to find time to climb up to the Sacré Coeur in Montmartre, where the temple of Mercury used to stand and where St Denis was beheaded.

But do not try to see too much. The best things in Paris are free or at least inexpensive. I bought a bread board for a few francs and with a soldering iron did a poker work drawing of the *Autoportrait par Hokusai* (1760–1849) from Japan, done in blood and ink. The latter is in the Musée Guimet in the Place d'Iena, which contains the most important collection of Indian, Indonesian, Japanese, Nepalese and Tibetan art in France.

Stop there and do not develop cultural indigestion.

LE MARAIS – PARIS

The most interesting part of Paris in my opinion is Le Marais (The Marsh). It reflects the style of France's leading families in the 17th century. This old aristocratic area stretches from the Place des Vosges westward to the Boulevard de Sebastopol, and from the Seine up to the Rue Réaumur and the Rue de Bretagne. Covering most of the

3rd and 4th arrondissements it consists essentially of seventeenth- and nineteenth-century town houses.

Charles V had his new palace Hotel St Paul erected here after 1358. Under Henry IV, the Place Royale (laid out between 1605 and 1612 and later renamed Place des Vosges) became the centre of court life.

During the eighteenth century, the Fanburg St Germain overtook it as the new elegant residential district.

Emptied by the revolution, and then confiscated by the State, the Marais' great houses were let out and converted into a honeycomb of small factories, storehouses and shops.

Restoration was commenced in 1962. On either side of the Rue des Francs-Bourgeois – 'Street of the outspoken middle classes' – lie a number of the finest houses. Hotel de Soubise was built between 1705 and 1709 by Delamair for the Prince of Soubise. The façade is decorated with sculptures of the Four Seasons – copies of the original by Robert Le Lorrains.

It now houses a Museum of French History with letters written by Jeanne d'Arc, the edict of Nantes, the diary of Louis XVI and Napoleon's Will. Another notable building is the Hotel Carnavallet. The place des Vosges, where Victor Hugo lived, now has the Musée Victor Hugo.

In the Rue de Rosier is the Jewish Quarter, where there have been recent bombings by the extreme Right party.

As I sat in a café after taking photographs, I had a glass of excellent French red wine. We are not yet a nation of wine drinkers to the same extent as the French. It is not necessary to ask for your red wine to be at room temperature (*chambré*).

When I went into a small café in the south of England and asked the waitress for a small bottle of red wine, she said, 'I'll have to go down to the cellar for it.'

'Never mind then, it will be too cold.'
'Oh that's quite all right sir, I can put on a pullover.'

LE MARAIS POITEVIN

Quite near La Rochelle is a unique part of France called the Marais Poitevin. We had met a Frenchman having coffee in Niort. As he had spent some time in Manchester – which we recognised from his English accent – he was pleased to converse in English and very generously conducted us to Coulon, about six miles distant, where we were able to take a boat trip along the canals.

The Poitevin Marshes are so called because of a twelfth-century word meaning near Poitiers. Sometimes the ancient dialect of the Languedoc is called *Le Poitevin*. The part near the sea is called *desséché* i.e. drained, and the landward part is *mouillé* i.e. marshy.

The canals have poplars along the banks as well as willows with silvery coloured foliage. The marsh dwellers – the *maraîchins* – use barges to carry their cattle and household needs. They navigate using a boat-hook called locally a *pigoulle*. Any Frenchman looking for a literal translation will not find it in the dictionary of the French language, *Petit Robert*, and certainly not in *Larousse*. But if I said in Doric 'It's a *gey tyauv*' – meaning 'It's a real struggle', I would not find the word Tyauv in the *Shorter Oxford English Dictionary*.

To return to the boatmen on the canals, they use also a short oar called a *pelle* – a shovel – to propel the barges which they call *yoles* – a word which, as one might expect comes from the country of canals, Holland, where it was first used in 1702. Beautiful though they are, the canals allow of no view, so that as in Finland, I enjoyed the visit but would not choose to live there permanently.

Like the Dutch, the canal dwellers have a milk cooperative which, if I may be allowed to use the word, churns out butter to add to the European butter mountain. As neither the French *maraichins* (marsh dwellers) or the Dutch see mountains from day to day, one can understand their attitude. The *maraichins* keep the skimmed milk to feed their pigs. They hunt otters, kingfishers, mullet, perch, carp and gudgeon. By using wicker traps, they trap shrimps and eels. We were told that in winter, game birds – duck, geese, snipe and herons abound. But communications with the locals is difficult – their dialect is difficult to follow, more so than the dialect of the Venetian gondoliers.

The *plainaud* – the man who lives on the 'levels' like the Pevensey levels – is typically broad shouldered, suntanned, with brown hair, sceptical and anti-clerical. Quibbling, quarrelsome and able to prove that four is five – he would make a good politician, but prefers life in his *bourrine* – a thatched cottage limewashed and snug in winter. They have a special costume called *maraichinage*. The verb *maraichiner* means a couple embracing sitting under a large umbrella to hide from prying eyes. Custom demands that the young lady at first rejects the advances, saying hesitantly, '*Y dirai au tchiuré (curé)* – 'I'll tell the priest what you're up to.' Finally, she consents and says, '*Fais tôt ce que tu veux mais vaque à ma coëffe*' – 'Do what you like, but don't mess up my hair-do.'

THE AUVERGNE – 1968

French people talk of the Auvergne as a hard and rugged land, lacking the ease and elegance of the south, so that it is not a popular tourist area. The landscape is volcanic, hilly in parts with in particular the famous Puy de Dôme which is more than 4,000 feet high, about the height of Ben Nevis in Scotland, which is the highest mountain in the British Isles. The name Auvergne derives from the Averni tribe, who strongly resisted Roman control of the area.

Vichy, associated in the minds of most people with mineral waters, as well as with its political rôle during the last war, is really a charming city, with perhaps more than its fair share of the elderly coming for spa treatment. There are some similarities in this respect with Eastbourne, which has never had spa facilities and no longer provides wheelchairs on the sea front, but is a haven for more mature folk. The most interesting town in my opinion is Mont Doré. It is a picturesque summer resort, a spa and a centre for winter sports.

The Puy de Dôme dominates the plain of Clermont-Ferrand. There is a toll road to the top with a gradient of 12%, usually closed from December to April on account of snow. It is possible to walk up from the end of the road to the summit where there are remains of a Roman temple to Mercury, a telecommunications tower and a magnificent panoramic view.

We visited nearby La Chaise Dieu, where the abbey church contains the celebrated *Danse Macabre*, 85 foot. mural, and Conques, a small fortified medieval town. It is also worthwhile seeing St Flour and its Gothic cathedral and the nearby Gabarit Viaduct built by Eiffel between 1872–1884, just before the Eiffel Tower in Paris; St Nectaire and Sales, all fairly near.

We watched a very impressive religious procession in Mont Doré, with purple-robed bishops and numerous clergymen in attendance. This visible hierarchy of the church reminded me of the story of a reception at Church House, Westminster. A waiter brought a tray of drinks to three clergymen – a vicar, canon and bishop. The vicar thought it prudent not to accept. The canon accepted hesitantly.

The bishop said, 'Alcohol! I'd rather commit adultery.'

Whereupon the vicar said, 'I didn't realise we had a choice.'

The church is often the object of kindly humorous anecdotes. A parson on his way by car to a neighbouring village to preach a sermon ran out of petrol. He called at a nearby cottage and asked an old lady for any form of receptacle to hold petrol. She could offer him only a chamber pot which he took to the nearby filling station.

As he was pouring the petrol into the tank of his car, two locals leaning on a bridge opposite said 'That's what I call real faith.'

Shortly afterwards, this old lady bought herself a pair of budgerigars. But a week later she returned to the shop and asked the manager how she could find out which was the male and which the female. The manager suggested that she should put a blanket over the cage and put out the lights. When she heard a sound, she should whip off the blanket and seize which bird was taking the initiative. This tactic was successful and she marked the male by putting a white ribbon round his neck. A few days later the vicar came to call on the old lady.

'Hello,' called out the budgerigar, 'caught you at it too, did they?'

My uncle, who was a country parson in the north-east of Scotland, had to conduct a funeral service one winter's day when there was deep snow. Eight bearers set off from the deceased's farm only a few fields away from the church. It was heavy work carrying the coffin through the deep snow, so they stopped from time to time for a rest to change bearers and have a wee dram from the hip flask.

When the eight red-faced bearers finally reached the church, my uncle asked 'Where's the coffin?'

The two groups of four bearers each thought that the other group had it. Not until a week or so later when the snow thawed and the whereabouts of the coffin became obvious was it possible to have the funeral service.

Although the Auvergne is described in tourist brochures as a country of spas and volcanoes and the natural fortress in the heart of the Massif Central, it has an important industrial city, Clermont-Ferrand. It is the capital of the Auvergne, a university town and the see of a bishop. Because local volcanic stone is used in the building of some of the houses in the old town, the name *Ville Noire* (Black Town) is sometimes used to describe Clermont-Ferrand.

The population is about the same as that of Brighton and it has France's largest rubber industry, as well as manufacturing, textiles, chemicals, food products and metal goods.

On another occasion, we stayed with friends, Dr and Mrs Desriac at a hospital at Montluçon, about 50 miles north of Clermont-Ferrand, and my daughter worked for a few weeks as a nurse. It is a pleasant town and has plenty of inexpensive accommodation for anyone wishing to stay there and visit the surrounding area.

THE ATLANTIC COAST (*Côte de l'Atlantique*)

This part of France with its fine sandy beaches and pleasant climate, had wooded dunes and a number of interesting islands such as the Ile d'Yeu, Ile de Ré and Ile d'Oleron. The islands are not hilly, and have been described as 'stranded marshes' – *marais échoués*. Because our daughter worked at Poitiers and La Rochelle, we got to know this area quite well. La Rochelle is a picturesque port with two towers, one at either side of the old port. The Tour de la Chaine is so called because a huge chain joined it with the Tour St Nicolas, so closing the inner port to invaders. The chain is now in the Museum of Orbigny.

The Lantern Tower – *Tour de la Lanterne* – is relatively new – not built until the fifteenth century – and has walls six metres thick at the base, contrasting with the elegant octagonal arrow on the carved foliated ornament on the pinnacle of the tower. The lantern, serving once upon a time as a guide for ships entering the port, is in the top. For a time, the Lantern Tower was used as a prison. The prisoners' graffiti – with similar motifs, but more elegantly drawn than those today – have survived from the seventeenth and eighteenth century and are protected by plates of glass.

If you go out on the balcony, there is a magnificent panorama of the harbour, the city of La Rochelle and the adjacent islands. At low tide, the sea wall built by Richelieu is visible.

Adjacent to the old port is the Clock Gate – *La Porte de la Grosse Horloge* – a gothic structure modified in the eighteenth century by the addition of a picturesque coping, comprising in the centre, a belfry which surmounts a dome and a lantern.

The Stock Exchange (*Hôtel de la Bourse*) has a façade adorned with sterns of ships and a variety of maritime trophies.

A couple of years ago we went to the Ile de Ré. Despite the GB plate, we were welcomed by the local people we met. They made no reference to the Duke of Buckingham whose fleet disembarked an army and laid siege to the capital St Martin in 1625, the 6,000 troops singing psalms before their assault.

Things were different in North Africa and Italy in that attacks were not in my experience preceded by psalm singing.

The islanders are celebrated for growing asparagus. At the western end of the island are the salt marshes – *les marais salants* – which seemed to cover about one third of the whole island. Other than at the salt marshes in Thailand, I had never been so impressed by the bare yet essential aspect of our civilisation. I had never been to the salt mines at Nantwich in Cheshire, and certainly not to Siberia, but I had read how much salt is prized in parts of the world where it is scarce.

As would be expected, there is a thriving fishing industry and oyster culture is now being developed.

All these aspects of life on the Ile de Ré lent themselves to photography and I took full advantage of the opportunities offered.

THE VOSGES – 1971

Relatively few tourists from Britain visiting France choose to go to the Vosges. There are English language editions of the Michelin *Green Guides* for Paris, Normandy, Brittany, the Loire and the Cote d'Azur which gives some indication of the more popular areas. Yet there is so much to be seen, such absorbing historical background and the local people are so welcoming, that visiting the Vosges is in many ways more interesting than visiting other parts of France.

We chose Orbey as a base, about ten miles north-west of Colmar, which is recommended as an excellent centre for the tourist. Orbey lies in the valley of the river Weiss, with numerous pathways, on the adjacent hillsides, which made an evening stroll most enjoyable. Our host at the Croix d'Or was genial and friendly.

We had food comparable to what would be expected in much more prestigious establishments. For the most part, the weather was good, but on a rainy day we went to nearby Colmar and spent some time in the Museum of Unterlinden. It is in an old convent and the name means 'Under the Lime Trees'. All around this area there is an appreciable German influence, with nearby villages called Kayserberg, Riguewihr, Sigolsheim, Kientzheim and Ammerschwihr.

The museum was built in the thirteenth century, and the ancient chapel of the Dominicans has the famous *Retable D'Issenheim*, a painting of the crucifixion by Grunewald dating back to the sixteenth century.

The most interesting building in the old part of the city is the Custom House built in 1480. It seems that they were able to extract rates and taxes with great thoroughness, even without computers. It must have been a more leisurely atmosphere than the London Stock Exchange, where highly intelligent young men working under considerable pressure for long hours burn themselves out in a relatively short time, unless they can unwind.

During a recent locum at a city medical clinic, I had to assess business executives. One very senior American head of a large organisation seemed exceptionally able, but rather tense, and the blood pressure reading was higher than it should have been. He said that he took no alcohol but admitted to smoking cigarettes.

'Have you ever seen a cow smoking a pipe?' I asked.

'No.'

'Or a cat puffing at a cigarette?'

'Never.'

He seemed offended when I said, 'They have more sense than to do that sort of thing,' but then smiled and admitted that I had made my point.

He knew the risks involved in smoking cigarettes and had for years worked solely as a statistician. I admitted that statistics could be used to prove many self-evident truths to be incorrect, but we agreed that cigarettes were carcinogenic. I told him about the traveller obliged in the course of his work to fly to all parts of the world. He had an obsessional fear of flying, but had to do so or he would lose his job. So he consulted a statistician to find out what were the risks of flying in an aircraft with a bomb on board.

'Give me a few days,' said the statistician, 'to consult the world's airlines and determine the risk.'

When the traveller came back to the statistician for advice he was told, 'Statistics show that there is only one chance in 2.5 million of you being in a plane with a bomb on board. But there is no recorded instance of there being two bombs on the same plane. So if you want to feel really secure, carry your own bomb.'

Then I got down to local affairs at the Eastbourne Town Hall. The town clerk explained to the town council that the death rate was 14.8.

When a councillor asked what this meant he was told, 'Fourteen dead and eight on the point of dying.'

As you can imagine, my thoughts were very far away whilst I contemplated the peace and quietness of the old Custom House in Colmar.

On another day we went to Strasbourg, the Capital of Europe, since 1949. It is claimed to be an incomparable city of the arts, built around its world famous cathedral. In the farthest parts of the world it is best known as the meeting place of the Council of Europe. With a population of about 250,000, it is relatively small in comparison with other cities less well known.

Undoubtedly, Strasbourg cathedral is quite magnificent. Victor Hugo, no mean critic, said, '*J'ai vu Chartres, j'ai vu Anvers, il me fallait Strasbourg*'. ('I may have seen the magnificent cathedrals of Chartres in Northern France and Antwerp, but what I must see is Strasbourg.') In a few sentences it would be impossible to refer to all the unique architectural detail, but the astronomical clock is probably the most popular curiosity. The seven days of the week are represented by chariots bearing various gods – these appear in an opening below the dial: Diana – Monday, then Mars, Mercury, Jupiter, Venus, Saturn, Apollo. Every 15 minutes two strokes are given, the first by one of two angels who frame the dial, the second by one of the 'Four Ages' who appear in front of the figure of death above the clock – the Infant strikes the first quarter, the Adolescent the second, the Man the third, and the Old Man the fourth. One must remember that the astronomical clock is half an hour behind normal time. At noon, there is a procession of apostles who salute Christ as they pass. Jesus blesses them during which time a cock, perched on the left tower, flaps his wings and crows three times.

The tourists gaze entranced – they reminded me of patients I had hastened to visit and were too engrossed gazing at Coronation Street to notice that I had arrived to save their very lives, perhaps.

The French seemed to venerate their elderly more than we do, although much less than the Japanese. When the model of the Old Man appeared in turn on the clock, there were nods and smiles of approval from those watching. Although it is 70 years since I read *Lettres de Mon Moulin* by Alphonse Daudet, I can still remember the passage in the chapter about old folks – Les Vieux. The frail old man was going into the village for a short walk and his elderly wife said, '*Tu ne rentreras pas trop tard; n'est-ce pas?*' Et lui, d'un petit air malin, '*Hé! Hé! ... je ne sais pas ... peut-être.*' ('Now don't be too long, will you?' receives the mischievous reply of the one time errant young man – 'I don't really know. Perhaps.')

One sentence from the Nobel prize winner Steinbeck's *Of Mice and Men* written in 1937 has stuck in my mind for 65 years. 'Take a really smart guy and he ain't hardly ever a nice fellow.' This could apply only to the smart alec opportunist and certainly all the 'smart guys' it has been my privilege to meet have been really nice fellows.

We were in the Vosges, if I remember rightly, and greatly enjoyed a trip along *La Route des Crêtes* – the Road of Crests – built by the French High Command in 1914–18 to improve military communications. It provides spectacular views of the *ballons* (a name given to the mountains of the Vosges), the lakes, the *chaumes* (thatched buildings which provide shelter in summer for the sheep), and the flowers. It is well worth while getting for only a few francs the beautifully illustrated 50-page book *Fleurs des Vosges* – Flowers of the Vosges. Muguets (*Maiglöckle*), lily of the valley, narcissi, orchids, clematis, aconites, anemones, potentillas, gentians and hundreds of other species abound. A botanist could find no better place to study the wide and infinite variety of flowers.

This is a wine growing region, where vines have been cultivated since the third century AD. The vine dominates the life of the country, the work and the festivities occupying more than 10,000 families of growers.

Water seems to be just as profitable. On the way north from the Vosges we stopped for a few hours at Contrexéville. Mineral waters have been used for remedial purposes from the earliest days of Greece and Rome. It is only during the past two or three decades that their sale in this country has become big business. More than 50,000,000 bottles are drunk each year, at a cost of several million pounds.

Many holidaymakers visiting France or Italy have continued to have a taste for bottled mineral waters after returning home. In our supermarkets, bottles of water from Contrexéville, Evian, Vichy, Badoit and Vittel are lined up beside a relatively small amount of native spring water, mainly from Malvern.

Some travellers abroad choose bottled water rather than drink tap water because of a mistaken belief that the purity of domestic water supplies is suspect. The choice of spring water in this country is thought to imply a degree of sophistication matching that displayed by connoisseurs of wine. Only a small number of those who opt for spa water do so because they believe that it will improve their health. It is unlikely that spa treatment will re-emerge solely because of the beneficial effect of the mineral content of the water. But the restful atmosphere, balanced diet, and congenial company are attractions which cannot easily be found elsewhere, except perhaps in relatively expensive health farms. So there are good prospects of a revival of interest in spas, similar to that existing in Germany and Russia at this time.

No one who has visited a spa town such as Contrexéville in the Vosges can fail to be impressed by the extent the local community has benefitted from the sale of bottled spring water. In this small town, a majority of the 5,000 inhabitants is employed directly or indirectly by the spa.

In the *charcuterie*, the proprietor explained that his son had a good job in the bottling plant.

'Go and see for yourself,' he said. 'Visitors are welcome every afternoon.'

So we went up the Rue de Lorraine to the *Usine d'Embouteillage* to see the bottling in progress. International recognition is ensured by the despatch of millions of bottles of Contrex, each bearing a label with a detailed analysis of the contents.

Jules Geraud, whose father we had met, urged us to taste the water. We did so, although we had already sampled the elixir at the *Pavillon des Sources*, after paying a small entrance fee. Visitors cannot, as happens in Buxton, carry off large plastic containers full of the water. Jules seemed to us to be an excellent ambassador, enthusiastic about the medicinal value of the product and anxious to make us feel welcome. He had a supervisory job and found time to explain his work. His wife, he told us, had a part-time job at one of the 17 hotels catering for the needs of those 'taking the cure'.

There are no indications at present of a lessening of the demand for mineral waters. Success has been achieved using a product free at source without expensive manufacturing costs and virtually without intensive sales promotion.

Advertising certainly pays handsome dividends. One particular brand of bottled mineral water is found in almost every hotel and bar in our country although I am not alone in thinking that it is not significantly different from other brands.

So we returned home, refreshed by the beauty of the Vosges and bearing samples of Contrexéville Water.

LES COLOMBIERS – 1973

A patient under my care in hospital had a niece, Madame Stassia Maillet, who came over from France to see her relative, and this led ultimately to a visit to her country house in a beautiful area of southern France, 30 miles north of Avignon near the Montagne du Luberon. The house, called Les Colombiers, was near Bonnieux in the Vaucluse area, and was surrounded by cherry trees in flower. Madame Maillet, a most kind and generous host, could speak Russian and expressed an interest in our visit to Kiev the previous year.

After flying from Heathrow to Marseilles, I was taken by a car sent to the airport by Madame Maillet and joined my daughter Rosalind. In spite of my shortcomings, they made me feel very welcome and Monsieur Maillet, who held an important position in the French Government, found time to take me to the Massif des Cèdres up in the Lubéron Mountains. There were magnificent views towards Avignon to the north-west and southwards towards the Mediterranean. During my stay there, I took a bus to Avignon on the Rhone. Avignon came to prominence in 1309 when Pope Clement V was compelled to leave Rome and seek refuge in France. There were seven Popes in succession who lived at Avignon until Gregory XI returned to Rome in 1377, and the town did not become a part of France until the French Revolution in 1791. The town walls, built in the fourteenth century, have 39 towers and 8 gates.

The Palace of the Popes is somewhat bare inside, but from the outside, with its massive towers and walls about 150-feet high, it looks like a feudal castle. After the French Revolution from 1810 until 1906 it was used as a barracks.

The best known feature of Avignon is the Pont St Bènèzet – the Pont d'Avignon – which was built between 1177 and 1185. It was partly destroyed in 1668, not, I was reliably informed, by the inhabitants, dancing on it – (you must know the song '*Sur le pont d'Avignon, on y danse...*').

In Avignon, the Musée Calvet, considered to be one of France's leading museums, has fine wrought-iron work and an admirable collection of pictures well worth seeing. During my relatively short stay in the Vaucluse I never encountered any British visitors – there is no *Green Michelin Guide* in English, but the Baedeker's *Guide to France* is excellent.

LOIRE – 1985

Romorantin – Lanthenay is about 25 miles south of Blois on the River Loire, yet seems remarkably free from the masses of tourists who visit the chateaux of the Loire. The *Green Michelin Guide* does not list Romorantin in its guide to the Loire, yet it is an excellent centre, and an enjoyable example of a French provincial town at its best. It is the capital of the Sologne, lively, bustling, with the River Saudre flowing through the centre, spanned by elegant bridges and flanked by old mills, timber-framed houses, and has large public gardens.

Nicholson's Guide to the Loire Region, written by Paul Atterbury, is an excellent little pocket book, easily the best guide to this part of France.

We had stopped for a time at Vendôme on the way south, where several branches of the River Loire flow amongst the streets. It has an excellent market day on a Friday, with a great selection of meat, fish, game, cheese and wine. Trinity Abbey (*Abbaye de la Trinitè*) has some fine sculpture on the west front, and stained glass which is exceptionally attractive.

We had previously visited Blois, so by-passed the town. Chateaux can be fascinating, but as one colleague said to me, 'Once you've seen one chateau you've seen them all.' However we did go to Valençay which was quite near and provided lots of interest on a rainy day. It was built in 1540 by Jacques d'Estampes, who had married a financier's wealthy daughter. Talleyrand, who started as Bishop of Autun under Louis XVI and was excommunicated by the Pope, had a somewhat chequered career being Foreign Minister from 1797 until 1807, and then quarrelling with Napoleon. Nevertheless, he was appointed ambassador to Great Britain from 1830 to 1834. He had bought Valençay in 1803 and used to host magnificent receptions. The animals in the park – llamas and deer – with the birds – cranes, peacocks, swans and flamingoes – interested me more than the chateau.

The city of Bourges is said to be at the centre of France, both geographically and historically.

The cathedral appealed to me more than any other cathedral I have ever visited. It is the widest Gothic cathedral in France and was built about the same time as Chartres Cathedral i.e. 1200–1260. No one travelling south of the Loire should miss visiting Bourges Cathedral – the first aspect which I found memorable was that I could park the car easily at the front door.

The sculpture, architecture and stained glass (circa 1220) are all exceptionally fine. We spent some time in the nearby Palais Jacques-Coeur, one of the finest Renaissance palaces in Europe. It was built in 1440 and has a great deal of exquisite carving.

St Leonard de Noblat, further west, was our next stopping place. In the *Red Michelin Guide*, a sign in red, of a bird, is supposed to mean a very quiet secluded hotel, but those who compiled the book could not have known that there was a wedding reception taking place on the same night as our stay. But, in reality, St Leonard de Noblat is a very attractive, small town with about 5,000 inhabitants, and an interesting church. It is well worth visiting.

Finally, if you are in this area, do not miss St Savin-Sur-Gartempe with its Romanesque church containing wall paintings, the finest being on the vaulting of the nave, illustrating the Biblical story of the creation onwards.

SOUTH-WEST

Travelling south from La Rochelle, the Ile d'Oleron, a popular seaside resort, is about 40 miles away. It is the biggest island in France after Corsica and has a large fish pond – *écluse à poissons* – which traps the fish as the tide goes out by having a series of grills, so that the fishermen can spear their catch.

By now, you are halfway to Royan, at the mouth of the River Gironde. It has been almost totally rebuilt after two terrible air raids in April 1945 – although it is now a beautiful fashionable resort, it took me hours to get rid of the thoughts of the carnage of 1945.

It is worthwhile going to the lighthouse – the *Phare de la Coubre* – to see the panorama. To the north, the Island of Oleron, beyond la Tremblade, to the south, La Pointe de Grave. It is more interesting to take the ferry over the Gironde, then to take the motorway, and go down to Mont de Marsan. It is the capital of the Marsan country and has a huge hippodrome, which has stables for at least 150 horses. No less famous is its rugby team. Unfortunately, we could not spend much time at Mont de Marsan as we had arranged to go on to Pau. Pau was discovered by British visitors in the 1820s, and has been popular with us ever since. Not surprising. The view from the Boulevard des Pyrenées is magnificent. The castle has an art museum with pictures by Tintoretto, El Greco, Rubens and Degas.

From Paul it is only a short distance – 25 miles – to Lourdes.

Apart from its exceptional religious importance, Lourdes is beautifully situated at the foot of the Pyrenées. It owes its fame to Bernadette Soubirous, who had a vision of the Virgin in 1858 and was guided by her to the spring which now supplies healing water to large numbers of pilgrims.

The largest church in Lourdes, St Pie-X, was completed only thirty years ago and can accommodate 20,000 pilgrims. It is somewhat of a paradox that my most vivid recollection of Lourdes is being involved in an accident when a reckless young man in a sports car drove into the side of my car, which at the time was almost stationary. He made off before I could catch him.

From Lourdes it is only about 30 miles south to the Cirque de Gavarnie, an imposing mountainous amphitheatre. It is rightly starred in all the guide books and no one who travels to Lourdes should leave it out of their itinerary. From the farthest point to which a car can be taken, it is possible to walk along a track beside a stream to the head of the valley. This takes about an hour and the view is exceptionally photogenic. A more leisurely approach is possible by hiring a mule.

The Grande Cascade, which has its source in Spanish territory, is the highest waterfall in Europe – more than 400 metres, well over 1,000 feet.

Travelling east it takes less than three hours to get to Andorra. This little principality is about the size of East Sussex, but has quite a number of differences. One is that there are no taxes levelled, because the income from advertising on Radio Andorra and the export of hydro-electric power meets all the government expenditure. Admittedly the resident population is only about 25,000 and they earn a great deal from tourism, but they seem to manage their affairs well. Mail is carried free of charge within Andorra, just as internal telephone calls in Moscow cost nothing.

Although the national language is Catalan, most Andorrans speak French or Spanish and a few speak English.

Carcassone, about half the size of Eastbourne, can be reached in an hour. It is the most complete example of a medieval fortified town to have been preserved intact. There are only two entrances to the town – the Porte Narbonnaise (Narbonne is 40 miles east on the Mediterranean) and the Porte d'Aude. A stroll along the ramparts is very pleasant and again, there is ample scope for the camera.

You can then choose to visit the Camargue or go north to Nimes and Avignon. The town of Arles is the gateway to the Camargue and the greatest touring centre in Provence. The Greeks settled there in the sixth century BC and it later became a Roman colony.

The amphitheatre is in many respects more interesting than the Colosseum in Rome or the Amphitheatre at Pula in Yugoslavia. Thermal baths were in use in the fourth century at the time of Constantine the Great – and there are scenes in Arles which were painted by Van Gogh. So, if you can't afford a Van Gogh, take a photograph. If I were to recommend further expeditions, it would lead to cultural indigestion – but Alphonse Daudet's Tartarin lived at Tarascon – and you could get there and back to Arles in a couple of hours.

But I have learned by bitter experience that one should not attempt to cram too much into a tour of France or anywhere else.

RABELAIS

(and a few anecdotes)

François Rabelais, born in 1483, is best known for his humanist philosophy expressed in works of richly inventive and often frankly coarse satire.

When Monseigneur Jean du Bellay, Bishop of Paris, was on his way to receive his Cardinal's hat in October, 1533, he suddenly became afflicted with terrible pains in the hips and buttocks, forcing him to stop at Lyon.

When a doctor was summoned, a youthfully middle-aged man appeared wearing a fur-edged robe and a skull cap decorated with a golden scarab, his merry face adorned with a clipped beard. It was, as you may have guessed, none other than François Rabelais, lecturer in anatomy at the hospital. Sciatica was diagnosed and a fee of ten gold louis demanded.

'Extortionate,' said the bishop.

'One louis,' said Rabelais, 'for the time and the balm.' 'Nine for being able to tell you the nature of your illness.'

When the bishop complained that the pills he had been given made him walk with a limp, Rabelais said, 'Well, that doesn't surprise me, there are two in your shoe.'

Rabelaisian stories may have appeared coarse and bawdy 500 years ago, but they are pallid in their imagery in comparison with the degenerate rubbish published today.

Quite often an incomplete knowledge of French can cause misunderstandings. A Lancashire man visiting Paris for the first time found a very thin inadequate mattress in his bedroom. He complained to the patron – the manager – '*Je veux dans mon lit un matelot*' – (a sailor).

'Ah, monsieur,' replied the manager, 'that is not possible.'

'Listen,' said the Lancashire lad, 'in my bedroom in England, I have two matelots.'

The manager replied in astonishment, '*Mon Dieu, quelle nation maritime.*'

Frank Muir claimed that he was unable to differentiate between a *piscine* (a swimming pool) and a *pissoire* (a urinal).

So when thanking his host in the south of France he said, 'You have a magnificent *pissoire* in your garden. I have used it on many occasions and found it remarkably warm, clean and relaxing.'

The housemaid at a country house got some petrol from the chauffeur with which she cleaned a pair of gloves. She was uncertain how to dispose of the petrol after use and poured it into the outside lavatory. Shortly afterwards the gardener entered the lavatory and stuck a match to light his pipe. The explosion which followed blew out the door of the lavatory. When the master of the house arrived, he found the gardener lying dazed just outside.

'Good gracious, George,' he exclaimed, 'whatever happened?'

'Oh, sir,' George relied, 'It must have been something I ate.'

A lady ill-versed in statistical argument had four children, but, even when pressed by admiring relatives, refused to have another. Why not? She had read that statistics showed that every fifth child born in the world is Chinese.

To return to the subject of housemaids in large country houses, a friend told me that he had been honoured with an invitation to have dinner with the Duchess of Dreck (This is the Jewish word for tripe).

On being asked how he enjoyed his dinner with the Duchess, he replied, 'If the melon had been as cold as the soup, if the soup had been as warm as the wine, and the wine as old as the chicken, and the chicken as tender as the housemaid, and the housemaid as willing as the Duchess, it would have been a very good evening.'

He decided to leave next day as he had planned a holiday abroad. On the way to the railway station, a school nurse smiled at him, as he was sitting opposite her on the upper deck of a bus.

'Why are you smiling at me like that?' said the man in a rather annoyed tone.

'Sorry,' said the school nurse in a loud voice, 'I thought that you were the father of one of my children.'

When he reached London, he spoke to a young Chinese girl he met in Regent Street 'Would you like to come up to my flat to see my stamp collection? You do look pretty.'

The Chinese girl replied, 'Philately will get you nowhere.'

Chinese is certainly a difficult language for us Westerners to learn. A Chinese patient was in hospital in a double room, very seriously ill. The other patient was British and didn't speak Chinese. So when the Chinese patient weakly said something, the Briton asked for help from an interpreter.

'What did he say?'

'You are standing on my oxygen tube.'

Misunderstandings abound in hospitals.

At a difficult caesarian section operation, the surgeon said to the anaesthetist, 'Is it a boy or a girl?'

A student nurse said, 'Let me see, I can tell the difference.'

Sometimes the patients are, not unnaturally, unfamiliar with medical terms.

'Excuse me doctor, but have you any anecdotes (antidotes) for a dirty tongue?'

'Please can I have some more of those oxyacetylene (tetracycline) tablets for that burning I get?'

Or the doctor can quite easily say something inappropriate on the spur of the moment. Asked by a patient who was an SRN why she should get a monilial vaginitis, I said I was not really sure – 'After all, that area is really a no-man's land.'

Sometimes, one comes across patients whose illnesses appear to be more imaginary than real. But I learned my lesson when I attended the funeral of one such patient. The inscription on the tombstone of the hypochondriac read, 'I told you so.'

It is easy to say the wrong thing quite unintentionally. For example, I said to one patient in hospital, 'We'll have you out of here quite soon, one way or the other.'

In Eastbourne, we have quite a number of retired people from London.

One such patient came to see me with a skin complaint, and said, 'I was being treated for this skin complaint where I used to live.'

'Acne?'

'No, 'ammersmith.'

A Welsh colleague told me about a young girl from Wales who became pregnant and did not want anyone locally to know about her condition. So she went to London and as she walked along, she saw a brass door plate with the name Dr Ralph Vaughan Williams.

When she rang the door bell, the housekeeper said, 'Sorry, he's gone to orchestrate the "Men of Harlech".

'And about time too,' said the girl.

There is an old Italian saying attributed to Giordanu Bruno (1585), '*Se non è vero è motto ben trovato*', which means 'If it is not true, it is a happy invention.'

When nurses' examination papers were scrutinised, there were several strange comments such as 'A blonde (bland) diet should be given to the patient suffering from gastric ulcer, as this usually helps to allay his suffering.' 'A pathologist is a man who sits on one stool and examines others.' On nightmares – 'A man had a nightmare that involved him being forced to eat shredded wheat all night long. When he awoke, half his straw mattress had disappeared.'

On incomplete abortions – 'the surgeon usually sends for the curate (curette).

'The successful candidate will be using her head – the only computer mass-produced by unskilled labour.'

At the prize giving, the late Sir Ludwig Guttman of Stoke Mandeville told of the anxious patient admitted to a double room at Stoke Mandeville hospital, the other patient, being an Australian, spoke Strine (Australian intonation).

'Have I come in here to die?' said the anxious man.

'No, yesterdie,' replied the Australian.

At another prize giving, Sir Graham Rowlandson, confined to a wheelchair, endowed with a brilliant intellect, and chairman of a hospital board, told how he attended an informal hospital meeting and as he was being carried downstairs and through the bar to his waiting Rolls Royce, one of the men in the bar was heard to say, 'Cor, that must have been some party they had upstairs.'

Another nurse wrote, 'Longer skirts will get rid of chilblains – and chaps as well,' and yet another wrote 'A woman's mind is cleaner than a man's because she changes it more often.'

THE WAR LEADERS

**FIELD MARSHAL ALEXANDER OF TUNIS,
Harold 1st Earl (1891–1969)**
After distinguished service in the First World War, Alexander held command in India. In the Second World War, he commanded the evacuation of British Forces from Dunkirk. After going along the beaches with a loud hailer, saying, 'Is there anyone still left?' he boarded a destroyer, being the last British soldier to leave France from the beaches.

He became Commander-in-Chief in the Middle East in 1942, and then as Eisenhower's deputy, directed the offensive that defeated the Germans in North Africa. He ended the war as Allied Supreme Commander in the Mediterranean and was subsequently Governor General of Canada (1946–1952) and Conservative Minister of Defence (1952–1954).

He latterly lived at Alfriston near Eastbourne in East Sussex and died in 1969 aged 77.

Liddell Hart, the distinguished war historian, wrote, 'He was a born leader ... but he might have been a greater commander if he had not been so nice a man and so deeply a gentleman.'

**FIELD MARSHAL HAIG,
Douglas 1st Earl (1861–1928)**
After service in North Africa and India, Haig in the First World War became Commander of the first army corps in France and later Commander-in-Chief of the British Expeditionary Force (1915). Haig has been criticised for the appalling losses of the Somme and Passchendale but his task was made more difficult by the lack of support from the Cabinet.

Haig commanded two million officers and men. A cavalryman with the finest attributes, he managed to enter the army, even though he was colour-blind. He was said to have had an uneven capacity for picking men, some of his subordinates being outstanding failures. Although highly intelligent, he was relatively inarticulate and not a good communicator.

By the end of the first battle of Ypres, there were 59,000 casualties. Winston Churchill described 1915 as a disastrous year. The names Somme, Arras and Passchendale were described as shadows over the name of Haig.

He had many obstacles to overcome. For example, in November 1918, the BEF had only 31,770 vehicles, whereas from D-Day 1944 until VE Day, 1945, Eisenhower had 970,000 vehicles, with a numerically smaller army, excellent radio communications and massive air support.

FIELD MARSHAL MONTGOMERY OF ALAMEIN, Bernard Law 1st Viscount (1887–1978)
In the First World War he became Commander of the Eighth Army (1942) and after the battle of Alamein drove Rommel back to Tunis and surrender (1943), an achievement that brought him enormous popularity. Having played a major role in the invasion of Italy (1943), he became Chief of land forces in the 1944 Normandy invasion. He helped plan the Arnhem disaster (Sept. 1944) but restored his reputation by pushing back the subsequent German offensive receiving Germany's surrender. After the war, he was Chief of the Imperial General Staff (1946–1948) and Deputy Commander of NATO forces (1951–1958).

Like some other brilliant and successful war leaders, he could be arrogant, ruthless and unwilling to admit his own shortcomings. Although involved in the planning of the catastrophic Dieppe raid, he seldom referred to the matter.

An American told me that the crossed swords worn as badges of rank were more suited to Montgomery than any other general because of his confrontations with other war leaders.

FIELD MARSHAL RUNDSTEDT,
Karl Rudolf Gerd von (1875–1953)
He was recalled from retirement at the outbreak of the Second World War, becoming in 1942 Commander-in-Chief in France. He held command in the battle of the Bulge (1944) and was considered by British military historians to have been Germany's most capable operational commander. He was captured in 1945, but his ill health secured his release. It is a measure of Adolf Hitler's charismatic leadership that he was able to control such a formidable personality as Von Runstedt.

ADMIRAL YAMOMOTO,
Isoroku (1884–1943)
Yamamoto was Japan's greatest naval strategist and commander. He was opposed to war with the USA because he believed that Japan would inevitably lose a protracted war against such a powerful opponent.

He started early in 1940 to plan the outstandingly successful attack on 7 December 1941, which crippled the US Pacific Fleet in Pearl Harbor.

His great contribution to naval strategy was his early recognition of air power and the development of long-range aircraft.

According to his biographer, he was betrayed by his own expertise into making one of the most colossal military blunders in his own country's and the world's, history.

MARSHAL ZHUKOV,
Georgi (1896–1974)
Marshal Zhukov was Deputy Supreme Commander-in-Chief of the Red Army for almost the entire war, taking a

major role both in planning overall strategy and in directing many effective campaigns in the field.

He was in personal charge of the defence of Leningrad (St. Petersburg) in November 1942 and of Moscow. Few people in the West today appreciate the immensity of the Eastern battlefront. By December 1941 the Red Army had had 5,000,000 casualties, 3 million prisoners and 20,000 tanks plus 30,000 guns destroyed.

Zhukov was imaginative and very successful, perhaps over-cautious, at the beginning of the war, but daring and decisive by the end.

In January 1942 Stalin refused the advice given by Zhukov, although Zhukov was ultimately proved correct.

The human cost of the Second World War was enormous, with a death toll of 50,000,000 of which 20,000,000 were Russian. Compare the US losses (300,000 killed) and the British (500,000 dead).

Interference by politicians accounted for millions of deaths – particularly in the case of Stalin and to a lesser extent Hitler. The damage done by Churchill and Roosevelt was small in comparison. Perhaps one of the least recognised politicians was President Harry S. Truman, who had the courage and strength of character to sack the megalomaniac General MacArthur, assessed by many military experts as the best General of the entire war and immensely popular with the American people.

STALIN,
Joseph (1879–1953)
He was born in Gori, Georgia on 21 December 1879 and named Joseph Vissarionovich Dzhugashvili. When he was a child his mother called him Soselo ('Little Soso') and he became known to his friends as Koba. Because his face was pock-marked he was nicknamed Pocky. He was considered to be a good swimmer.

His father, a cobbler, Vissarius (Beso) Dzhugashvili, was a morose and frightening drinker. Stalin escaped from the home environment and married 16-year-old Keke.

By this time, Lenin, eight years older than Stalin, became his role model. Lenin was the son of a state councillor, in rank corresponding to a general. Stalin was described as Lenin's left leg.

Koba was an ineffective speaker with a muffled voice, slow speech and a Georgian accent. Even his enemies feared his secretive character, his subtle sarcasm and his rough outbursts of anger.

He had had a rather disturbed childhood and was later subject to physical abuse in an Asiatic jail, suffering beatings from the warders, living in filthy conditions with total deprivation of rights.

Eisenhower described Stalin as benign and friendly, barely five feet tall, with white hair in a crew cut, wearing a white jacket that made him look like an elderly sommelier. He considered that Stalin was a man whose sigh could mean torture or death.

'One may smile and smile, but be a villain.'

I have been fortunate to meet many interesting personalities in my life. Among them, I remember...

LORD HAILSHAM – died October, 2001
Many years ago, when the present Lord Hailsham, as Quintin Hogg, was MP for the Combined Universities, his father Lord Hailsham, who lived at Carter's Corner, Hailsham, in Sussex, became ill with pneumonia. Quintin Hogg phoned the family doctor, Dr Keith Robson of Herstmonceux, expressing concern at his father's health and of course at the same time naturally realising that if anything should happen to the old man, he, Quintin Hogg, would

succeed to the title and lose his seat as an MP for the Combined Universities. However, Dr Robson prescribed penicillin and the old man recovered. Some months later he had yet another attack of pneumonia and once again Quintin Hogg phoned to enquire, to be told that a further recovery had taken place. Ultimately, however, the old man died and Quintin Hogg succeeded to the title.

He continued to live at Carter's Corner. On a Saturday morning, when he was first Lord of the Admiralty and was down for the weekend in Sussex, one of the farm workers injured his hand in a tractor at Hailsham. Lord Hailsham bundled him into his car and drove him straight into St Mary's Hospital, which was relatively quiet for a Saturday morning. The patient had to be taken to the operating theatre to have the hand attended to and Lord Hailsham made it clear that he would not leave the building until he was satisfied that his farm worker had been properly attended to. So I invited him into the Medical Staff Room. Like so many politicians, with a brilliant intellect, he was a voluble and articulate conversationalist. He told me that the work at the Admiralty was very demanding and time-consuming, saying that he would have to get back that evening to get on with the paperwork. I suggested that if ministerial responsibilities were so heavy that it might be better if ministries could be divided up as, for example, having a Minister of Agriculture and a Ministry of Fisheries, rather than one Minister of Agriculture and Fisheries.

To this suggestion, Lord Hailsham replied, 'My boy, there are insufficient people in the House of Commons with the requisite intelligence to exercise ministerial responsibility.'

This remark and similar comments in Parliament did not endear him to his colleagues. His autobiography, entitled *The Door Wherein I Went*, makes interesting reading.

LORD SHAWCROSS – October 1964

As Sir Hartley Shawcross, the present Lord Shawcross came to be widely known and recognised as a brilliant lawyer when he appeared as prosecutor in the Nuremberg trials.

Now retired, he lives at Cowbeech, East Sussex. Some years ago, one of his resident staff, Mrs Miller, had a stroke, requiring her admission to hospital under my care. She made good progress, but remained disabled to some extent and we had to discuss her future care. Having been resident in the Shawcross household for many years, she had no home to go to on leaving hospital.

Knowing this, Lord Shawcross wrote, in his own hand, a most kindly and thoughtful letter, explaining that although the lady had given years of excellent service, it was not *practicable* for her to return to Friston Manor. We were able to place the patient in a home for elderly disabled persons, where she was very happy in the company of others of her own age and state of health.

Like so many eminent and brilliant men, Lord Shawcross was kindly and considerate. One of his intellectual colleagues was the late Lord Cohen of Birkenhead and Lord Shawcross gave a marvellous eulogy at a meeting of the Royal Society of Health in Eastbourne.

Sadly, Lady Shawcross died following a riding accident at Friston. She had been President of the Friends of the Samaritans in Eastbourne and was greatly missed.

SIR KEITH JOSEPH

The day before Sir Keith Joseph, then Secretary of State Department of Health and Social Security, was due to visit Eastbourne to study hospital resources available for the elderly, I was asked by a highly respected colleague in practice at Herstmonceaux to visit an elderly man. The patient was confused, incontinent, malodorous and living alone, apart from a variety of pets, in a shack at the bottom of a field. It was impossible to carry out an adequate clinical examination under these conditions so I arranged immediate admission to hospital in Eastbourne.

Promptly at the agreed time next morning, the ministerial limousine carrying Sir Keith drew up at the front door of the hospital. He jumped out, brushed aside any suggestion of detailed introductions to the welcoming party saying, 'I've come to see the patients – they are the most important people here and all of us are here to serve them to the best of our ability'. He then went directly to the male acute geriatric admission ward and spoke to the first patient nearest the door – who happened to be the man I had seen the previous evening.

'How are you, my good man?'

'Thieves have broken into my country mansion and stolen over a million pounds worth of art treasures.'

'Indeed – indeed'.

I turned to our chairman and said, 'If this sort of dialogue goes on all day he won't know what is fact and what is fiction'.

The chairman's reply was, 'If he's been in the House of Commons for fifteen years, and can't tell the difference, I don't think much of him as a politician'.

LORD MONCKTON OF BRENCHLEY

In 1959, Lord Monckton and his wife moved to Folkington Vicarage near Eastbourne. Viscountess Monckton was known to our hospital committee chairman, the late Dr Gordon Masefield, as both were members of the Regional Hospital Board.

During a meeting of the committee of the Friends of the Hospitals, Lady Monckton phoned to seek medical aid from Dr Masefield, as she had no other medical contact in the area. He felt that, as a retired psychiatrist, he should not deal with the situation, so asked me to go. Taking a nursing sister with me I went to see Lady Monckton and treated an acute ear infection.

A few weeks later, Lord Monckton needed help, so I returned to their home, prescribed a simple remedy and said that, whilst it was a privilege to treat someone who had done so much for others – he was then chairman of St George's Hospital, Hyde Park Corner and chairman of the Midland Bank – it would be more appropriate if he were to see a 'proper doctor'. Shortly afterwards, I received the following letter:

Midland Bank
22 May, 1959

I am writing a word to thank you so much for all the trouble you took for me last week-end. I am relieved that the culture showed no signs of growth and I have had a word with my doctor as you advised. I realise that it was unprofessional to worry you and am grateful though ashamed.

Yours sincerely
MONCKTON OF BRENCHLEY

EARL MOUNTBATTEN OF BURMA

Earl Mountbatten was born in 1900, the younger son of Prince Louis of Battenburg, who later became First Sea Lord.

As a consequence of anti-German sentiment, the family name was changed to Mountbatten in 1917. His career is well-known and he was Captain of the Navy Polo Team. In 1955 he realised his ambition by becoming First Sea Lord and Chief of the Naval Staff – the first time a father and son had both become professional Head of the Navy.

Each year, at Annual Representative Meetings of the British Medical Association, there is a lunch or dinner for past and present officers of the Royal Army Medical Corps.

We were greatly honoured when Earl Mountbatten agreed to speak at our dinner at Millbank Military Hospital. He drove himself from Broadlands in Hampshire, and with the utmost courtesy shook hands with the 30 or 40 members present. After dinner he spoke quietly and most interestingly about a variety of topics, including medical treatment he had received following polo accidents in the Mediterranean. Then he drove back to Broadlands.

Like every civilised person, I was nauseated by his cold-blooded murder.

DAVID CHARD – died 13 January, 1997
A Welshman, he joined the army in March 1940 and was posted to a heavy artillery regiment with six-inch guns from the 1914–18 war, pulled by commandeered civilian lorries. The officers' transport was Brighton taxis. The men wore civilian clothes, with old army great-coats. Later David joined the 15th Regiment of Royal Field Artillery going to Egypt and Syria. His regiment landed at Taranto, later being part of the 78th Division with the yellow Battleaxe emblem.

At 7.00 p.m. on the 11th April, 1945, one month before hostilities ended in Italy, he was a battery observation post sergeant on a Sexton Tank. When the Germans made one of their last desperate counter-attacks, David dismounted to guide the tank driver into a sheltered position between two farm buildings. As he did so, an 88 shell landed, wounded him in seven places, including the left ankle and calf, but most importantly in the back, at the level of the 10th to 12th thoracic vertebrae. He retained the shell fragment, about one ounce in weight, which severed the spinal cord, leaving him paraplegic – paralysed permanently from the waist downwards, a condition he endured for nearly 60 years.

As is the experience of others with a sudden paraplegia,

he felt as though his legs were weightless, and levitating. He recalled that it was raining heavily at the time, that he was initially attended by a number of magnificent Polish infantry who took him to a forward medical unit from which he was transferred to Rimini where he arrived at 3.00 a.m.

It was not until the 21st June 1946, 14 months after being wounded, that he ultimately got to the Spinal Injuries Unit at Stoke Mandeville. He remained there until 1948, after which he came to the Chaseley Home for Paraplegics in Eastbourne, where he met his wife Audrey.

In spite of his entire life being altered by what had happened in Italy, both Audrey and David developed a great liking for the country and had many close friends in Italy who so admired David that he was given a flat at Gravellona near Lake Orta, adjacent to Lake Maggiore, where they could both live in perpetuity. Although they have visited Italy many times and stayed at Gravellona for periods of time, David was happier when he was near Stoke Mandeville, whose care undoubtedly saved his life. It requires little thought on the part of the reader to realize the immense part Audrey has played and I regard it as a great honour to be counted amongst their many friends.

It is not surprising that amongst the guests at his birthday party many distinguished Italian friends made the long journey in his honour.

From May 1948 until 1964, he worked at the Dental Estimates Board at Eastbourne, until the late Sir Ludwig Guttman advised him to retire on health grounds. He was then aged 47, had only one kidney, multiple kidney stones and severe high blood pressure.

David had a totally different personality to my own. He never complained to me, was invariably cheerful, optimistic, and with the requisite intelligence to have had an outstandingly successful career were it not for his war injuries.

JIMMY SAVILLE

It was the custom of the Eastbourne Hospitals' Sports and Social Club to elect a Beauty Queen each year. In the year that Jimmy Saville was appearing at the Congress Theatre, we asked him if he would crown the queen and he readily agreed to do so.

At about 10.30 p.m., after we had selected the queen for the year, he arrived following his performance, at the Social Club party. Now it so happened that the previous beauty queen had departed, taking the crown with her. So we had to hastily make a cardboard crown, decorate it with gold paint, and paste on pieces of coloured glass to represent precious jewels.

Jimmy Saville appeared, dressed in a velvet suit, with long blond hair, carrying a tape recorder to preserve all that was said. It was soon obvious to me that beneath the velvet suit and blond hair, was a highly intelligent quick-witted man, who had exceptional talent.

So he took the cardboard crown and said, 'I crown this beautiful girl with this golden crown, studded with rubies, emeralds, sapphires, diamonds and even Double Diamonds.'

After I had thanked him on behalf of the club, I said that he must be tired after a demanding stage performance, followed by the ceremony at the club. Would he be able to get to bed soon?

'Yes, my brother is outside the building with a dormobile, I shall be asleep in five minutes and when I wake, we shall be in Leeds.'

He was going to work voluntarily as a porter at St James's Hospital, Leeds next day. A most remarkable man, who has done a great deal of good for disadvantaged people. I admire him greatly.

MIKE YARWOOD

In his early days, Mike Yarwood agreed to officiate at our annual fête, and appeared to me to be a little anxious for someone well-accustomed to public appearances. The reason was that his wife was going to have her first baby in St Mary's Hospital. He was a most charming man, who quickly endeared himself to everyone present and confirmed my impression that to get to the top in show business requires outstanding talent and a pleasant personality.

TOMMY TRINDER
Tommy Trinder gave a most amusing speech when he opened our hospital fête, so I felt rather nervous when I had to thank him for doing so, but he quickly put me at my ease and by his presence ensured that the fête was well-attended and a great success.

DR JOHN BODKIN ADAMS
It is seldom that an Eastbourne doctor can avoid being questioned by a medical colleague of mature years in any part of the world about Bodkin Adams.

A Belfast graduate, he was a strong muscular type, who competed in the Isle of Man TT Motor Cycle races, and, when he came to Eastbourne in 1922, did his rounds on a motor cycle. He practised with a group of doctors, but was a loner. Soon after I started in Eastbourne, he used to telephone me at the hospital, asking if I would complete cremation certificates. He did not wish to introduce other practising doctors to the family of a deceased patient in case the family might change their allegiance. He knew that I was not in competition for private patients and that I was only too pleased to earn an extra guinea.

Later I was to have some misgivings about my actions when Superintendent Hannam of Scotland Yard came to my office with a sheaf of certificates which I had signed in good faith.

Early in 1948, when there were frequent meetings about the imminent National Health Service, he drove me to a meeting in Tunbridge Wells, and talked about the possibility of my joining his practice, but I was already actively involved in the work at St Mary's Hospital, so declined.

About a year later, I was invited by one of the Eastbourne surgeons, Lawrence Snowball, to assist at a perineo-abdominal excision of rectum at the Esperance Nursing Home.

Adams was the anaesthetist and I was mildly surprised, even in the year 1948, when one of the nuns wheeled a tea trolley into the operating theatre. Whilst Snowball and I sweated at the operating table, Adams lowered his face mask and had tea from a large silver teapot, with a plentiful supply of meringues and cream cakes.

It was whilst I was having lunch at an official function with the Chief Constable that his deputy Superintendent Seekings informed him that Adams had been arrested. The story made headlines around the world – I was introduced at a meeting in Germany many years later as a doctor from Dr Adams's town.

When I passed the examination for the Institute of Advanced Motorists he phoned to congratulate me – he was himself a member of the Institute – and drove me to a road safety discussion at Battle. During the journey he talked incessantly about how the authorities had 'got it in for him', and seemed genuinely to believe that he had been victimised. It was only after his death in 1983, at the age of 84, that, with the threat of libel removed, books began to proliferate on the subject. Lord Devlin wrote, 'Dr Adams was not a sensible man; he was on the contrary a stupid, obstinate and self-righteous man. He was also an indiscreet and incessant talker.' With these sentiments I agree, except that I would substitute 'less intelligent than others' for the word stupid.

When a medical colleague, the late Dr A.G. Emslie, was fishing for salmon in a Scottish loch, he sought the advice of his ghillie – a Highlander who attends a sportsman at fishing.

'I've been trying for hours without success, and I've used all the best flies – any suggestions?'

'Try this one, sir. It's a "Bodkin Adams" – a sure killer.'

MISUNDERSTANDINGS

Misunderstandings may arise from:

Impaired hearing
 Did the TV weather presenter say 'Rain will become more expensive in southern Scotland'?
Literal translations
 We must ferret out the fox (from the Chinese film *Crouching Tiger, Hidden Dragon*)
Different spellings of words which sound alike
 'My son spends most of his time fencing.'
 'Has he attended a school for swordsmanship?'
 'No – just building trade courses at the college of further education.'

Verdi's *Rigoletto* – Meanwhile the villain Scarpia continues to press his suit.

'Have you seen Stravinsky's *Rite of Spring*?'
'Yes – but my musical tastes differ. In fact, it seemed somewhat avant garde, by my standards, quite wrong.'

After Cervantes had been wounded at the Battle of Lepanto in 1571 he had a crippled left hand – hence his nickname 'El Manco' – a left-handed person. But manco also means defective or faulty – a word not be any means apposite to Cervantes.

Polo mints are said to be the only contraceptive pill approved by the Pope – because they are holy...

WORDS OF THE GREAT

Field Marshal Lord Ironside, Chief of Imperial General Staff 1939, on Field Marshal Lord Gort VC DSO and bar, MC Commander of British Expedition Force 1937–40:
'Completely out of his depth as CIGS.'

Pownall on Ironside:
'Quite unsuited to be C-in-C on a modern battlefield. Would be all right bush-whacking or knocking the Middle East about, but he is not intelligent – not enough so as to deal with a first class enemy.'

Ironside on Ironside:
'I am not suited in temperament to such a job nor have I prepared myself to be such.'

Pownall:
Called Ironside and Churchill 'The Crazy Gang'; made ironic comments on 'those major strategists' – Winston and Ironside.

Ironside:
Found Churchill's seesaw changes of mood hard to cope with, described the frequent rambling discussions of chiefs of staff like a lot of children playing a game of chess.

FIRE-EATERS

Not until about 1677 was the question of the proof of man against fire looked at from a scientific standpoint. Studies were carried out by the physician Dodart, a member of the French Academy of Sciences, provoked by feats being performed at that time in Paris by an English chemist named Richardson. Experiments had been carried out by an Italian physician and chemist, Sementini, using various substances to protect the human skin against fire including sulphurous acid, alum, soap and powdered sugar.

Fire-eaters have always been very popular on the vaudeville stage. They cause flames to dart from the fingers, sometimes producing a brilliant flame from the mouth without putting anything inside the mouth cavity, but simply blowing the flames from the fingers.

Eaters of burning tow may form a little ball of material which they tightly compress and then light, allowing it to burn up almost entirely.

Some only pretend to drink paraffin, held in an iron ladle, which is then lit. They dip a spoon into the blazing oil, which, when held for a moment in front of the open mouth, gives the impression of fire eating.

A more dangerous and realistic demonstration was witnessed recently in the Square Willette, near the Sacré Coeur in Paris. The performer invited passers-by to throw a one franc coin on to a chalked Cross of Lorraine on the paving stones. When the cross had been covered with francs, he proceeded to fill his mouth with paraffin, which he blew outwards and upwards, lighting the jet with a burning rag held on a stick in his hand.

HOBBIES

GLASS ENGRAVING

Glass engraving has many attractions. It requires no previous skill or experience, costs very little – one can buy glass beakers, jugs, vases, tumblers, beer mugs and wine glasses at bric-a-brac stalls very cheaply – and needs the minimum of equipment – initially just a sharp-pointed steel stylo and a pattern to glue on to the inside of the glass. For example, a timetable for French railways, available free at railway stations has a design of the Cathedral of Notre Dame, which can be cut out, pasted inside the glass vessel and outlined with the stylo. A paper bag provided to hold postcards of Lincoln has a design of Lincoln Cathedral, which again can be pasted on the inner surface of the vessel. Lettering, old or new, can be collected from newspapers and magazines to enable the initials of a friend to be engraved on the glass. If one is more ambitious and can afford to purchase an electrically-powered engraving drill work can be done more quickly and precisely. These drills are not expensive and a dental surgeon may be willing to give the glass engraver his old dental drills which he would otherwise throw out. Useful domestic objects such as jam jars, can be engraved with the words, Tea, Sugar, Coffee and so on which cannot be rubbed off with washing, but can be covered with a self-adhesive label if another use for the glass container is thought to be desirable.

Patterns of flowers, animals, trees, mountain scenery are obtainable from glass-engraving firms for a few pence so that the hobby can be pursued by anyone who has reasonable eyesight and a steady hand. Of course, it takes a great deal of time and patience to reach the standard one associates with the professional glass engraver. However, even the beginner can obtain a great deal of satisfaction from his or her early work, which is generally appreciated as useful. A personalised object can be a most acceptable gift. There can be few hobbies so easily done, at so little cost, and provide useful and acceptable gifts.

There is a most useful publication on this subject entitled *Engraving Glass – a Beginner's Guide* by Boyd Graham.

PEWTER

The enthusiast invariably regards his interest as superceding all others. Not everyone has read the book by W.R. Lethaby published in 1893 entitled *Lead Work*.

The author says that tin and lead were responsible for the early fame of Britain, as they brought here the Phoenician traders and had doubtless much to do with the consequent Roman occupation. Certainly Cornish tin was mined and exported to Rome via Gaul overland, as well as by ship, and the invaders were already proficient in the uses to which it could be put.

Pewter is an alloy of tin with lead or copper, antimony and bismuth. Britannia metal, also an alloy of tin, copper and antimony was introduced in the late eighteenth century by James Vickers of Sheffield (1769). Is it or is it not pewter? A large proportion of American pewter today is Britannia metal. Thomas Danforth Boardman was the first to experiment with the new alloy in America and began to produce teapots around 1805 and 1806. By using Britannia metal, it was possible to make a far greater range of objects more cheaply and in fashionable styles. Because it was easier to mass-produce and therefore cheaper than the original pewter, this led sometimes to poor design and low standards of production. The terms 'hard metal', 'white metal' or 'French metal' came to be synonymous with

Britannia metal. If you see the letters EPBM stamped on a pewter-like object, you will know that it is electroplate on Britannia metal.

On a number of occasions, I have challenged dealers who have claimed that a Britannia metal object is genuine pewter. Some do not appear to know the difference – or say so. It is difficult for them to respond to such a challenge. Rather like the schoolboy who was asked, 'Have you not done your homework or are you just plain stupid?' How does he answer?

Many medical instruments used to be made in pewter; castor oil spoons, bleeding bowls, syringes, and eye baths.

The earliest written record of an organisation for the regulation of the pewter craft in England was made in 1348, when the pewterers of London petitioned the Mayor and Aldermen of the City for ordinances framed for the protection of the workmen from fraud and unfair competition and for the guarantee that a high standard of workmanship and an adequate quality of metal should be maintained thenceforth.

A copy of the original petition, transcribed in Latin and Norman French, remains in the City archives and there is a copy in the records of the Worshipful Company of Pewterers of London. Amongst the objects listed were pots, salers (salt-cellars), porringers (*esquelles* – a word not to be found in the Petit Robert *Dictionnaire de la Langue Français*), platters, cruets, chrismatories (sacramental annointing vessels) and other things that are made square or cistils (ribbed). 'Vessels of Pewter' (vessele desteym) had to have one hundredweight of tin to 22lbs. of lead (lay or ley metal).

Misdemeanours such as theft under the value of ten pence had to be made good, a second offence was punishable and the offender was put out of the craft if he committed a third offence.

No one was to be 'so daring as to work at night' lest poor light resulted in unsatisfactory standards of workmanship.

From 1503 onwards, pewter marks were mandatory.

Various kinds of drinking vessels were amongst the commonest pewter articles made during the past four hundred years. In 1482 there are references to 'Tanggerd Pots' and Stope Potts i.e. Stoop or Stoup Pots. Some of the spelling then was of the same calibre as the graffiti spelling on our walls in 1987.

Measures for beer were made as early as 1351. The popular term 'Tappit Hen' is the familiar title bestowed on an essentially Scottish type of wine measure. The word 'tappit' is derived from the French *topynet*, a French measure of capacity. A *topette* is the French word for a small long straight bottle. The true 'tappit hen' is a measure of one Scots pint capacity, a Scots pint being equivalent to three English (or Imperial) pints.

Candlesticks, salt cellars and spoons were often made of pewter. Our word salt cellar is derived from the French *salière* meaning a salt holder, so it is rather like talking of a traumatic injury to speak of a salt cellar. But we have all heard uneducated doctors talking about traumatic injuries. Medical language has not changed much since the early days of pewter – I have heard a surgeon say 'Pass me the bleeding bowl' when he has no intention of embarking on blood letting. Nor did the surgeon make himself understood when he said to the medical student 'What is the bleeding time?' and got the answer 'Ten past four, sir.' Surgeons are often misunderstood. An eminent and confident consultant surgeon said to the patient pre-operatively: 'Your operation is *bound* to be successful. Textbooks describe a 90% mortality and my last nine patients who had the same op have all died.'

Of course, patients can easily misunderstand advice

given. A woman frequently visited a hospital out-patient department for the follow-up of an innocent heart murmur, reported *The Lancet*. She had four children all by the same father, with whom she had been living for many years, although she had remained unmarried. The rather puzzled physician asked what she had against matrimony and was told, 'When I was sixteen I saw the professor who told me that I had a heart murmur, and although I could lead a normal life in all ways, I must never get married.'

Fairly simple wording can avoid some misunderstandings.

A geriatrician whose hobby was bird watching was out on the moors in Scotland and said to the ghillie, 'Are there any octogenarians in this part of the country?'

The ghillie replied 'Only twa – and we shot them both.'

A rugger player with a dislocated shoulder was taken to the local cottage hospital and put in the next room to a woman in labour.

'You're making a terrible noise,' said the nursing sister, 'more than the woman in labour.'

'Maybe,' said the rugger player, 'but she doesn't have to have it put back.'

Sometimes even the Aberdeen newspapers write articles which are open to misrepresentation. Recording the anniversary of Napoleon's death in 1821, the *Aberdeen Press and Journal* notes, 'His doctors thought he had been laid low by chronic hepatitis brought on by the damp climate in exile in the Isle of St Helena. Medical opinion has subsequently diagnosed everything from gastric ulcers to stomach cancer. Although the liberal doses of arsenic he took might not have helped his condition, there was not much wrong with him when his coffin was opened 19 years later.'

Better to be non-committal, like the politician giving a

ministerial reply as recalled by Lord Hume of the Hirsel, 'That may well be. If so, what then?'

Surgeons however are usually pretty forthright.

When the uncertain young anaesthetist said during the operation, 'God help me,' the surgeon overheard and said, 'I will not have any unqualified assistant in my operating theatre.'

When my colleague asked for an aperitif, the waitress seemed rather surprised and said, 'A pair of teeth?'

At a Church of England Synod at York, Bishop Stockwood told how he lost his false teeth during an ordination retreat in the diocese of Lichfield. Stockwood rummaged high and low in the rambling Georgian house opposite the cathedral, but could find them nowhere. A fortnight later however, when he donned his episcopal finery for an ordination, he discovered them with a resounding thud, lodged inside his mitre.

'It gave an extra bite to my sermon,' he said.

We were talking about collecting pewter as a hobby. It is quite surprising how little it costs for a piece of old pewter lying in a junk shop in a small town not frequented by tourists. If cleaning is required, use no more than warm soapy water and polish with a soft duster.

If you are looking for pewter abroad, remember that in many European languages there is no distinction between pewter and tin. In France, look for *étain*. Tenn and zinn mean not only tin but also pewter.

If you have spent hours studying the question of lead-free petrol, you may hesitate about using pewter which contains a small amount of lead, but in fact you are unlikely to use a pewter utensil for eating or drinking nowadays. The alloy in use today contains no lead. In the United Kingdom, new pewter tankards which are often given as presentations and are inscribed contain 94% tin, 4% antimony and 2% copper or bismuth.

If you are interested in old pottery, the book by Salmon, published in Paris in 1788 *L'Art du Potier d'Étain* is beautifully illustrated. The study of pottery can be just as satisfying as purchasing pottery. There is plenty to be seen in the Victoria and Albert Museum in London, the Rijksmuseum in Amsterdam and the Landesmuseum in Zurich. In the Rijksmuseum, the pewter collection is named Heemskirk, after the captain of a Dutch ship which foundered in 1596 at the island of Novaya Zemlya, in the Soviet archipelago off the north coast between the Barents and Kara Seas. The ship contained pewter candlesticks, flagons and salt containers.

In a pewter inkstand made in the late eighteenth century, there is an upper drawer for wafers with a lower drawer pierced for pounce i.e. powdered pumice, for use as blotting paper. But even ink has now gone out of fashion. When I asked for a bottle of ink in a vast emporium in the basement of a five-star hotel in Detroit, the girl did not know what it was.

'We have only ball-point pens,' she said.

Pewter styles differ in different countries and it is possible to identify the country of origin after a fairly short study of the subject.

Now there is some beautiful modern pewter, but the original pewter still has the greater attraction for many of us.

THE CLARINET

In spite of never achieving proficiency in playing the clarinet, it has given me considerable pleasure. Like many children, I had a recorder whilst at school and, being a Scot, a bagpipe chanter. It was unfortunate that when I decided to take clarinet lessons about 25 years ago, I was heavily committed and under stress with hospital and committee work, so did not devote sufficient time to practice, even though I had an excellent teacher in Mr Harry Cooper.

About eighty years ago, Wilhelm Altenburg wrote *Die Klarinette*, and later Agostino Gabucci produced *Origine e Storia del Clarinetto*. When Geoffrey Rendall published, *The Clarinet – Some notes on its History and Construction*, it was widely acknowledged as being the work of the leading authority on the clarinet in this country, probably in the world. Adam Carse's *Collection of Musical Wind Instruments* published in 1951 first stimulated my renewed interest, although at the time it was impossible for me to take lessons.

Not many people appreciate that there is only one essential difference between a clarinet and a saxophone. The former has a cylindrical bore, the latter a conical bore. Both can be made of wood or metal, can be straight or curved with an upturned bell, and can vary in length from 14 inches to nine feet.

Most players prefer a clarinet made of wood or ebonite (vulcanite). It is frequently made in five separate pieces – the mouthpiece, the barrel, the body in two separate pieces and the bell, so as to make the clarinet easily portable when dismantled. In fact, there is much to be said for making the body in one piece as was the custom in early clarinets. A double-bass player becomes accustomed to carrying a large instrument in buses, trains and aeroplanes. There seems to be no real need to adhere to the usual five piece clarinet.

With the passage of time, attitudes change.

At the conclusion of the General Strike in 1926, a Labour government was in power, with Ramsay Macdonald as Prime Minister. Fleet Street asked for a photograph of the Cabinet outside 10 Downing Street, to which they readily agreed.

In 1926 photographs were taken using a magnesium flash gun and the camera lenses were covered with caps. The doyen of the press photographers brought half a dozen of his colleagues, lined them up in a row opposite the Labour Cabinet standing in Downing Street, each member of the Cabinet wearing the traditional cloth cap.

When the senior photographer explained to his colleagues that one magnesium flash would suffice for all the photographers, he said that he would set off the flash when he gave the order to his colleagues to remove their lens caps.

'Caps off,' he shouted.

To a man, each member of the Labour Cabinet removed his cap.

The same photographer told how he was given an assignment to photograph the King of the Belgians, then staying incognito at Claridges. As an aside, it has always seemed odd to me that the King of the Belgians is so called, whereas we do not speak of the Queen of the British, or the King of the Spaniards. There is, as some of you may know, a pub called the King of the Belgians in Huntingdon.

The press learnt that the King of the Belgians liked to take an early morning stroll before breakfast, so the photographer arrived at Claridges at 7 a.m. When the King came out, the photographer suggested that he could do no better than take a short trip on the then open-top London bus to see the sights. All went well, the King was delighted and the photographer got all the pictures he wanted.

When the conductor said, 'Fares, please,' the King, as is the custom with royalty was carrying no money, so the photographer paid the fare, with one of the only two coins he had in his pocket.

Later the same day, he went to Chequers to photograph Ramsay Macdonald on a flag day. The prime minister stepped outside, stood beside the old lady with the collecting box, but he too had no money in his pocket. So the photographer gave Ramsay Macdonald his last coin, and took a photograph as the coin was being placed in the box.

Then he set off by bus to return to Fleet Street with his photographic scoops.

'Fare, please,' said the conductor.

The photographer had no money so he said to the bus conductor, 'Sorry mate, I can't pay. I've given my last two coins to the King of the Belgians and the Prime Minister.'

To return to the clarinet, the enthusiast can develop what a doctor calls tunnel vision – he cannot conceive of anything relevant but his own clarinet.

The famous professional musician R.S. Rockstro writes, 'It may be admitted unreservedly that machinery of any kind on a wind instrument is an unfortunate necessity.' Did he not start with a recorder or even a tin whistle as I did?

In fact, most clarinettists play other wind instruments and indeed many are highly proficient pianists and equally at home with the violin.

It seems that reed instruments have fascinated musicians at least as early as the beginning of the third millennium. Egypt may be the country of their origin. There is a Sardinian *launeddas*, a Basque *alboquea*, a Slav *brelka*, and a Welsh *Pibgorn*.

In India a snake charmer uses a *pungi*. The French *chalumeaux* is illustrated in the *Encyclopaedia* of Diderot and d'Alembert in 1767.

The extent to which I have been Anglicised by living in Eastbourne for the past 55 years is shown by the fact that it is a clarinet rather than bagpipes which keeps me happy.

CHAMPAGNE

At the Abbey of Hautvillers, south of Reims in France is a

carving of Dom Perignon, a blind Benedictine monk, and 'father' of Champagne. He was born there in 1634 and was cellarer of the abbey for almost 50 years until he died in 1715.

Rarely has a man established himself in history so firmly, and this was partly due to his extraordinary expertise, and his association with Claude Moët, who was born in 1683, lived near Hautvillers in the Vineyard Village of Cumières and cultivated his vines in the Marne Valley.

In 1743 he founded the House of Moët, where he was followed first by his son Nicolas-Claude (1719–1792) and then by his grandson Jean-Rémy (1758–1841).

After the French Revolution, the Abbey of Hautvillers and its vineyards were acquired by Moët. In 1832 Jean-Rémy Moët handed over the house to his son Victor, and his son-in-law, Pierre-Gabrielle Chandon. Since then the company has been known as Moët and Chandon.

The quality and delicacy of Moët and Chandon Champagne is derived from Black Grapes (*Pinot Noir*) from the Montagne de Reims, Pinot Meunier from the Vallée de la Marne and White Grapes (*Chardonnay*) from the Côte des Blancs.

The harvest is the culmination of a year of careful tending of the vines. Between late September and mid-October, when the grapes are fully ripe, hundreds of pickers gather the harvest, and tip their baskets into osier trays supervised by experienced old women who have been picking grapes for most of their lives.

The best grapes go into bigger osier baskets called *Caques* (kegs).

In Epernay, the heart of the vineyards, the juice is rapidly separated from the pulp using traditional presses. It then descends into the *cuves de débourbage* ('Clearing vats') beneath the presses, where it remains for a few hours to allow the solid matter suspended in the juice to settle.

The clear juice which leaves the *cuves de débourbage* goes into oak casks or stainless steel vats to be transformed into wine by its first fermentation, *le bouillage* – a local term not found in the Petit Robert *French Dictionary*, meaning a form of distillation although in fact there is no distillation. For several weeks the wine must be kept at a constant temperature of 20°C during which time the 'must' (new wine) bubbles and sings with the action of the yeasts it contains.

When the *bouillage* is complete, the wines are cooled before being 'racked' to remove any deposit.

After the first fermentation, the directors and *chef de cave* prepare the *cuvée* – the vintage by blending the new wines from a great number of growths of the three different grapes.

After the *prise de mousse* – bubbles which cause the wine to sparkle, the bottles remain *sur lattes* – on racks – in cellars to mature over a number of years. It is only with time that champagne can achieve the incomparable delicacy and taste for which it is renowned.

During the second fermentation a sediment forms which must be removed. The bottles are placed *sur point*, neck downwards, in *pupitres* – lecterns. Then every day over a period of several months *remeurs* – removals – manipulate the bottles causing the sediment to slide down until it rests on the cork. After several months, the neck of each bottle is frozen, after which, the sediment, imprisoned in a small pellet of ice, is expelled by the process known as *dégorgement*. Afterwards, each bottle is topped up with a small quantity of cane sugar previously dissolved in old wine (*liquer de tirage*).

So a very dry (*brut*) or dry (*sec*) wine is produced and so also may be a sweet or slightly sweet wine.

The bottle is then sealed with a new cork, held in place by the familiar wire muzzle.

Moët and Chandon are proud to show their Visitors'

Book containing the names of Napoleon, Wellington, Metternich, Petain, Nikia Khrouchtchev and many others, including Madame Pompadour.

There are of course many famous names in the Champagne world – Veuve Cliquot (the Widow), Pol Roger, Heidseick, Mumm and many others. Only a real connoisseur can differentiate when he tastes a champagne.

That the founder Claude Moët was able to pass on to his son and grandson the incomparable assets was partly due to the different approach to death duties in these days. In recent years in this country a wealthy farmer made a will leaving £100,000 each to his three sons. Four and a half years later in July, after lunch, he was found dead in bed. Naturally the sons were very concerned – not least because they had spent a lot of money in riotous living in anticipation of the inheritance. At that time, a period of five years had to elapse before the entitlement could be received.

So they put the body of their deceased father reverently in the deep freeze. In the following January, six months later, they removed the body and laid it on the bed. When the doctor was called, he said that he would have to ask for an inquest, as he had not seen the patient for at least six months. After a post mortem examination, the coroner certified death as being due to natural causes.

After the sons had returned home to celebrate the successful outcome, the doctor called and said, 'I've called to ask about the post mortem findings, because the stomach contents included fresh strawberries and one does not usually have these in January.'

'Ah,' said the eldest son, 'you should know that we have a very good deep freeze.'

Apart from the standard bottles available, there are different sizes with delightful Biblical names, for the most part, named according to the number of standard bottle equivalents.

Magnum	2
Jeroboam	4
Rehoboam	6
Methuselah	8
Salmanazar	12
Balthazar	16
Nebuchadnezzar	20

Champagne will never be cheap. The work involved in its preparation makes this obvious. Yet ten years ago nearly 200,000,000 bottles were sold.

If you are buying a bottle of champagne, do not choose one with the words *Methode Champenoise* on the label. If it has, the bottle has come from elsewhere. Unlike all other French wines, champagne does not have to state its *Appellation Contrôlée* status. The one word 'champagne' is enough.

The most important and revealing item of information on a champagne label is the CIVC, or *Comite Interprofessional du Vin de Champagne*, registration code which is printed in minute lettering. The first two letters of the code are the key to the champagne's origin.

Unless you are a really genuine connoisseur, do not get too worked up about the vintage years. Many so-called experts cannot tell the difference.

History abounds with apposite comments about champagne – a true luxury. Champagne at cocktail parties taken in moderation need not blunt the wits.

When Lady Margot Asquith met Jean Harlow on one such occasion, Jean Harlow said, 'Your first name and my surname sound alike.'

'Yes' said Lady Margot, 'but the really significant difference is that my first name ends with the letter T.'

Asquith had a fine turn of wit at times, but was subjected to the customary back-biting which occurs in Parliament.

R. S. S. Crossman – Tricky Dicky as he used to be called in BMA circles – said of James Callaghan, 'He is not just a schemer ... he talks to me in the friendliest manner, and then fights me ruthlessly behind my back.'

Another parliamentarian was once described by the brilliant *Daily Telegraph* Parliamentary Correspondent, Mr Godfrey Barker, in this way, 'He got up with the lapel-clasping piety of a nightclub proprietor recently admitted to Holy Orders.'

Tasting champagne is widely regarded by the afficionados as one of the great pleasures of this life. For my part, I would prefer to be witty as I enjoy making people laugh. But I fear that this will never happen.

GAUGIN

Paul Gaugin, the French Impressionist painter, was born in Paris in 1848. After five years at sea, he became a stockbroker in 1871, painting only as a hobby. His early works were influenced by the Impressionists with whom he exhibited between 1881 and 1886. He became a full-time painter in 1883 and moved to Brittany in 1886, where he developed a style called Synthetism. He did so along with Émile Bernard (1868–1941). The visual arts counterpart to the symbolist literary movement, synthetism sought to express an idea or emotion through formal correspondences of line and colour. It was also known as *cloisonnisme*, since its use of rich unmodulated colour contained within thick black contours resembled *cloissoné*.

Cloisonné (French; partitioned) is a technique of decorating metal surfaces with polychrome enamelwork – the art of decorating metal surfaces with coloured glass that is fused on to the metal. There are three kinds – *Cloisonné* – *Champlevé* and painted enamelwork. The technique of painted enamelwork involves painting powdered wet enamel all over the metal before firing. Painted enamel is particularly associated with Limoges (fifteenth and sixteenth centuries) and England (eighteenth century).

In such paintings as *Vision after the Sermon*, which is in the National Gallery at Edinburgh, he illustrated what he meant by symbolism.

In 1873 Gaugin married a Danish girl whom he met in Paris, Mette Gaad, a straightforward practical, narrow-minded and hyper-conventional woman. They had five children in ten years.

He visited Martinique in 1887, and stayed with Van Gogh in Arles in 1888. Seeking the inspiration of a primitive civilisation – *toujours la politesse* – he left his wife and he moved to Tahiti in 1891 where the symbolism in such paintings as *Nevermore*, which can be seen in the Courtauld Institute in London, was influenced by native superstitions.

Gaugin is noted also for reviving the art of woodcarving (*La sculpture sur bois*). He wrote to his favourite daughter, Aline, 'With lots of pride, I finally got lots of energy and I have willed to win.'

He painted Breton peasant girls, women in Martinique. Painting became the all-consuming interest in his life whilst he was a stockbroker. A consultant surgeon with a brilliant record and outstandingly successful in his processional work plans to retire early to devote himself to painting. It is addictive. The conversation has been envisaged as a brutal crisis, a sort of coup de foudre, an impulsive act, or as Somerset Maugham calls it 'a spell.'

Although Gaugin was a symbolist, deep inside he made fun of the movement and its dogmatism. Monfried said that Gaugin approved of Verlaine, saying ironically at the Café Voltaire, 'Oh bother (or similar expletive); they annoy me these 'cymbalists'.

In Martinique, he was asked 'Do you seek a wife?' A Maori woman brought him a tall, slender vigorous child of 13, with whom he lived until his death. I like best his last work 'Breton Village Covered by Snow' painted in 1903 and now in The Louvre.

PAINTING

My interest in painting originated when I started bringing home prints as souvenirs.

Until a few years ago, I was convinced that I was quite incapable of painting, until I met a Mrs Mary Alford who was not only a trained artist but an enthusiastic teacher.

She insisted that I should and could paint, so that I was quite overcome by her persuasive approach.

Now I enjoy watercolour painting and prefer to paint rather than, for example, watch television, unless there is an exceptionally good programme. Active rather than passive activities promote good health and I find it easy to become totally absorbed in painting, however inadequate the finished product. Merely trying to paint has made me much more aware of the brilliance of the old masters. Even a poor amateur footballer is better able to judge the skill of a top professional than someone who has never played the game.

Heightened sensitivity brings immense pleasure to these with even a rudimentary knowledge of the subject. The steady increase in attendances at National Trust gardens has grown side by side with more people taking an interest in their own gardens.

I now get much greater enjoyment out of going to an art gallery than formerly. The fairly recently opened Musée d'Orsay in Paris seemed more fascinating than the Louvre or the National Gallery which I had visited years ago.

I like to think that my paintings are gradually improving and urge the reader to give painting a trial – so many people I have got to know recently who have just started painting after retirement and got immense satisfaction from their efforts, encourages me to try to persuade you to do the same.

'A man should hear a little music, read a little poetry, and see a fine picture every day of his life in order that worldly cares may not obliterate the sense of the beautiful which God has implanted in this human soul.' Göethe.

OBITUARIES

It is a satisfying experience to help grieving relatives by describing the high regard for the lost one by former colleagues, and having a tribute published by the British Medical Journal.

It is helpful to have some knowledge of the BMA and to study the advice given by former editors. Give the truth about a rounded human being, with all achievements. Avoid clichés, such as 'work was his hobby', 'marks the end of an era', 'will not see his like again'. It is better to avoid phrases such as 'caring for patients with skill and compassion', 'supremely confident'. Nothing is gained by describing the foibles – this can be really upsetting for the family.

Since submitting an obituary notice in 1974 a further 30 of mine have been published. In every instance the opinion of members of the family have been of paramount importance. Self-written tributes are sometimes rather deprecating – 'O wad some power the giftie gie us, to see ourselves as ithers see us'.

During the past fifty years in Eastbourne the need to be sympathetic and not sycophantic has been learned.

After outliving all my former associates of 1947 I am no longer sufficiently understanding or knowledgeable to describe the contribution which has been made by the new generation.

FAMILY LIFE

Oliver Goldsmith wrote that the man who married and brought up a family did more service than he who continued single and only talked of population. Not every man has the good fortune to have a loving and devoted family and I know with absolute certainty that I could not have achieved anything of value or even be still alive were it not for my family.

My wife has had to tolerate my absences, lateness, eccentricities and support me in so many ways that I marvel she has not deserted me years ago. My elder daughter Elizabeth has been equally tolerant, and is happily married with two grown-up children, Mark and Angela. Her husband by his own efforts and technical skill created a lovely house which was originally built by a Dutch civil engineer employed to deal with the drainage of the Somerset levels, not dissimilar to the problems encountered and successfully handled in the Low Countries.

Mark graduated from Hull University and worked for a car leasing firm in Florida. He is now co-partner in a garage in Exeter. Angela graduated from Leicester University and is currently living in Turin, where she is marketing director of an Italian firm which manufactures bathroom fittings and exports them worldwide.

We naturally enjoy their visits to Eastbourne, and took them to see the Newhaven Fort, with its underground passages, gun ports, and ammunition stores. It was during the coal strike and they had watched the television coverage as well as the children's programmes.

So when I asked Mark if he was interested in the fort, he was most enthusiastic. Angela on the other hand, said that she felt like McGregor – cold and bored.

It is difficult for me to write about my own family, but I

do feel that 100 years ago, Robert Louis Stevenson expressed how I feel much more adequately than I could myself,

'To be honest, to be kind – to earn a little and to spend a little less, to make upon the whole a family happier for his presence, to renounce when that shall be necessary, and not be embittered, to keep a few friends, but those without capitulation – above all, on the same grim condition, to keep friends with himself – here is a task for all that a man has of fortitude and delicacy.'

Because my younger daughter is a teacher of English as a foreign language, I have, for some years, felt that I ought to try to improve my meagre knowledge of French and have joined the Eastbourne Branch of the *Foyer Français*.

Most people from other countries appreciate it if one tries to speak even a few words of their language. This can lead to difficulties as when for example a Minister of Education, over confident about his knowledge of French, addressed a group of French students visiting London by saying, '*Pendant trois années j'étais dans le cabinet*,' not realising that French people think of a cabinet as a toilet.

Another misunderstanding arose when, at an official function, an Elder Brother of Trinity House sitting next to a French guest said, '*Je suis un frère ainé de la Trinité*' ('I am an elder brother of the trinity') to which the astonished Frenchman replied, '*Mon Dieu – quelle situation.*'

Sometimes we take our desire for racial equality a little far. The Race Relations Act was passed with good intentions but when a medical colleague, also from Aberdeen advertised for a Scottish cook as he enjoyed porridge for breakfast, he was summoned for publishing an advertisement implying racial discrimination.

CONCLUSIONS

Many readers of these autobiographical notes may by now be akin to the peer who dreamt that he was speaking in the House of Lords and woke up to find that he was. If what has been written has induced sleep, then a benefit has been conferred on the reader.

It has been my good fortune to live an active life, to have received help and support from friends more intelligent and industrious than myself, to have enjoyed good health and to have survived beyond the age of retirement.

It is beyond my capacity to thank all those whose kind support has enabled me to help others less fortunate than myself.

My life has been pervaded by a sense of inadequacy which has been a driving force. My greatest enjoyment has been meeting others in all walks of life in different countries, with different attitudes towards life.

The British of course, are noted for their tolerance. One of the reasons why I hold our royal family in high regard is that they refrained from violent reactions when Earl Mountbatten was murdered. Her Majesty behaved in a most exemplary way when an intruder entered her bedroom. This episode of intrusion into the Queen's room made the British security services the laughing stock of the world – I have always felt embarrassed when asked to explain how such a thing could happen in Great Britain.

In no other country but Britain would those responsible for security have been let off so lightly. If the monarch had asked that the Home Secretary and Commissioner of Police be dismissed, this would have been accepted in other parts of the world as a natural reaction.

My admiration for the courage of many severely disabled persons whom I have been privileged to meet is boundless.

Likewise, I admire some politicians, especially Margaret Thatcher, whose ability and stamina is astonishing. We in Eastbourne were fortunate in having an exceptionally kind and industrious Member of Parliament, of great ability, whose work earned the respect and affection of the entire community – Mr Ian Gow.

Ian Gow was murdered by the IRA outside his home, the Dog House, Hankham, East Sussex. Within days of being elected MP for Eastbourne he asked me to take him round the Eastbourne hospitals and later invited my wife and me to lunch at his home.

Just as the BMA made a major error in opposing the introduction of the National Health Service, so our government made a vastly greater mistake in embarking on the Falklands War.

It may be a sombre thought but is of fundamental importance – it is my firm belief that we shall never experience a nuclear war.

BIBLIOGRAPHY

Alanbrooke Field Marshal Lord (Editor: Danchev and Todman) *War Diaries 1939–1945*, Weidenfeld & Nicolson
Beckett Frank, *Prepare to Move With the Sixth Armoured Division*, 1993
Cloake John, *Templer Tiger of Malaysia*, Harrap
Ellis John, *Cassino-The Hollow Victory*, Sphere
Fraser Sir David, *Life of Field Marshal Erwin Rommel, Knight's Cross*, Harper Collins
Majdalany Fred, *Cassino – Portrait of a Battle*, Longman Green 1957